P9-DND-275

Is Your Body Trying to Tell You Something?

OTHER BOOKS BY CARMEN RENEE BERRY

When Helping You is Hurting Me: Escaping the Messiah Trap
(Harper & Row, 1988)

Loving Yourself as Your Neighbor
A Recovery Guide for Christians Escaping Burnout & Codependency
(with Mark Lloyd Taylor)
(Harper & Row, 1990)

How to Escape the Messiah Trap: A Workbook
(HarperSanFrancisco, 1991)

Are You Having Fun Yet?
How to Bring the Art of Play Into Your Recovery
(Thomas Nelson, 1992)

girlfriends: Invisible Bonds, Enduring Ties
(with Tamara Traeder)
(Wildcat Canyon Press, 1995)

Who's To Blame?
Escape the Victim Trap & Gain Personal Power in Your Relationships
(with Mark W. Baker)
(Piñon Press, 1996)

Coming Home to Your Body:
365 Simple Ways to Nourish Yourself Inside and Out
(PageMill Press, 1996)

The girlfriends Keepsake Book: The Story of Our Friendship
(with Tamara Traeder)
(Wildcat Canyon Press, 1996)

Is Your Body Trying to Tell You Something?

Why It Is Wise to Listen to Your Body and
How Massage and Body Work Can Help

CARMEN RENEE BERRY

PageMill Press
A Division of Circulus Publishing Group, Inc.
Berkeley, California

Is Your Body Trying to Tell You Something?
Why It Is Wise to Listen to Your Body and How Massage and
Body Work Can Help

Formerly titled **Your Body Never Lies**

Copyright © 1993, 1997 by Carmen Renee Berry

All Rights Reserved under International and Pan-American Copyright
Conventions. Published in the United States by PageMill Press, a division of
Circulus Publishing Group, Inc. No part of this book may be reproduced in whole
or in part without written permission from the publisher, except by a reviewer who
may quote brief passages in a review; nor may any part of this
book be reproduced, stored in a retrieval system, or transmitted in any form
or by any means electronic, mechanical, photocopying, recording, or other, without
written permission from the publisher.

Publisher: Tamara C. Traeder
Editorial Director: Roy M. Carlisle
Copyeditor: Jean Blomquist
Jacket Design: Gordon Chun Design

Typeset by Cragmont Publications, Oakland, California
Typographic specifications: Text is set in Adobe Minion 11/14;
chapter titles are Minion Display

Printed in the United States of America

LIBRARY OF CONGRESS CATALOGING-IN-PUBLICATION DATA
Berry, Carmen Renee.
    [Your body never lies]
    Is your body trying to tell you something? : why it is wise to listen to your body
and how massage and body work can help / Carmen Renee Berry.
        p. cm.
    Originally published in 1993 by PageMill Press under the title:
Your body never lies.
    Includes bibliographical references.
    ISBN 1-879290-11-1
    1. Touch—Therapeutic use. 2. Massage therapy. 3. Mind and body therapies.
I. Title
RC489.T69B47   1997
615.8'22—dc21   96-43499
                                                                     CIP

Distributed to the trade by Publishers Group West
10 9 8 7 6 5 4 3 2
97 98 99

DEDICATION

To Roy M. Carlisle

for restoring my hope
in the healing power of shared love.

CONTENTS

ACKNOWLEDGMENTS

I want to thank the many people who have touched me, physically and emotionally, in such a way to support my healing and growth.

First, I want to thank Dr. Joan Overturf, who astutely recognized, many years ago, that my body had been ostracized from the rest of me. At her urging, I took the risk of trusting my body, a risk that, at that time, seemed sheer folly. Looking back, I can trace much of the healing and contentment I now enjoy to her body-based wisdom and insight.

I have benefited from the nurturance of a number of talented massage and body workers. I especially want to thank Jean Yano, my first body worker. With her quiet, firm and nurturing touch, Jean introduced me to my body, a gift for which I will be forever grateful.

In addition, many body workers have contributed to my progress, including:

Charles Swan	Timothy Bennett
Jasmine Bailey	Cheryl Hewitt
Martin Nunez	Joe LaPorta
Claudette Renner	Martti Makinen
Ray Swartley	Rosa Sanchez
Mandy Stephen	Blanca O'Neal
Carlos Rivera	Eva Parvianen

I want to express particular gratitude to Carolyn J. Braddock, body worker par excellence. Her unique approach to body work unlocked secrets my body had held for far too long. My life has been changed due to the way she helped me honor, listen, believe, and follow the wisdom of my body.

I am grateful to my body work support group: Susan Latta, Virginia Frederich and Kate O'Sullivan. The group provided a safe place for me to put my body-based, nonverbal experiences into words. Their candid sharing about their experiences greatly contributed to my ever-growing understanding of the body, of spirituality, and of the healing power of touch.

My current therapist, Dr. Paul Roberts has also helped me further articulate and benefit from my experience with massage and body work. He has become an "attuned" companion with whom I explore and expand my capacity for intimacy. He has truly created a safe place in which I grow.

I want to thank my parents, Dr. David and Ellen Berry, for years of support and affirmation of my professional development. Their never-wavering belief in me undergirds my sense of purpose.

Through the many days of writing this manuscript, especially the weeks when I literally disappeared from sight, I want to thank my friends. I relied heavily on their patience and supportive, though sometimes bizarre, phone-machine messages and faxes, to press on to completion. These long-suffering, ever-supportive friends include Bobette Buster, Joel Miller, Pat Luehrs, Rene Chansler, Cathy Smith, Bob Parsons, Gail Walker, Bob Myers, Irene Flores, Alex LaBrecque, Dale Ryan, Dan Psaute, Rick Fraser, Jim Kermath, Mark Baker, Stephen Smith, and Daryl Quick.

I also want to thank Noreen Naughton, Joann Connors, Pauline Krismanich, and Ann Chamberlin of Immaculate Heart Community for their continued support of my writing and for providing me with a place to hide away to work on the manuscript.

A special thanks goes to Alicia Porter, my assistant and friend, for the many ways she contributed to this manuscript. She spent hours in the library locating needed materials, returned phone calls when I was hiding away with my computer, and got me to laugh at myself when I was taking it all a bit too seriously.

I have relied heavily on the support, wisdom, and outrageous humor of my booking agent and friend, Lynn Barrington. I am grateful to have benefited from her talent, her creativity, and her endless energy. Thanks, Lynn.

Working with the PageMill Press family has been a delight

and a welcomed change from traditional publishing. I am grateful to Tamara Traeder for her wise leadership, for including me as a viable member of the publishing team, and for making me laugh a lot during our phone conversations.

And last, but not least, I appreciate Roy M. Carlisle, who has worn so many hats in the project that we've all lost count. He believed in this project from it's inception, and it's not an overstatement to claim that the book would not be published without him. In addition to his contribution to this book professionally, he has, through his friendship to me over the years, supported my personal exploration of body work. In honor of his tireless commitment to me, I dedicate this book to him.

Professional Consultation

Special thanks to my colleagues who have assisted in the development of this book through professional consultation. Each of these individuals have made a unique contribution in the fields of psychology, theology, medicine, and/or body work. I deeply appreciate the helpful suggestions, the provision of bibliographical resources, and the intellectual challenge I received from the following:

Carolyn J. Braddock, M.A.
Roy M. Carlisle, M.A.
Virginia Frederich, M.F.C.C.
Jim Kermath, M.Div.
Alexander LaBrecque, Ph.D. Candidate

Susan Latta, M.F.C.C.
Constance Lillas, Ph.D.
Joel Miller, M.D.
Kate O'Sullivan, M.F.C.C.
Dale Ryan, Ph.D.
Catherine Smith, Ph.D.

PREFACE

Authors often compare writing a book with giving birth. Since I have not given birth to a flesh-and-blood baby I can't be certain the analogy applies, but as I write this preface as the last task in this project, I feel very much like I imagine a new mother. Utterly exhausted yet thrilled to have my child finally in my arms.

Putting words to my experience, as a recipient of massage and as a body worker, has been much more difficult than I imagined when I first conceived of this book. Much of what goes on in a body work session is non-verbal, even pre-verbal. Translating these experiences into words that communicate the depth and power of the moment in a credible manner has been a challenge. I pray that I have been able to convey this reality clearly and believably.

Another challenge has come from my religious beliefs. I am a Christian with a vibrant, personal relationship with God. While my relationship with God has been and continues to be the ground for my life, I have been extremely disappointed by how I have been impacted, and at some points damaged, by the Christian church. Based on what I believe is a misinterpretation of scripture to support an anti-body, anti-touch bias, I was taught not only to disregard my body but to view my body as the source of "sin." Whenever my body was included in Christian spiritual disciplines, the body was viewed as part of the problem, not a source of guidance or communication with God. I now utterly reject this heretical notion.

I believe God led me to explore massage and body work as a legitimate and healing spiritual discipline. Massage and body work are much more to me than methods of stress management or therapeutic healing. They are avenues by which God and I communicate, disciplines as valid as any traditional approach to spiritual growth such as prayer, scripture reading, worship, confession, or participating in the eucharist. I believe that all of the benefits of massage and body work, including increased health and vitality, enlarged capacity to enjoy intimacy, appropriate expression of feelings, and healing of past trauma is possible because of the spiritual nature of touch. For massage and body work to be genuinely helpful we must be able to relax, confident that we are safe and protected. This safety is possible, I believe, because God does in fact participate in this process and provide us with spiritual protection.

Learning about massage and body work was spiritually challenging for me. I could find no "christian" body workers or massage school when I started my journey many years ago. Those interested in massage and body work often work from an eastern or new age perspective, spiritual paradigms to which I do not ascribe. In addition, many who shared my Christian perspective or professional mental health background, viewed massage and body work as spiritually dangerous, sexually provocative, professionally foolhardy and down right "flakey." In spite of these challenges, God encouraged me to continue in my exploration through the transformation I experienced as my body was honored through touch.

I do not overtly discuss my Christian beliefs in this book with the intent to offer what I have learned to people from all faiths and perspectives. Nevertheless, I want to take this opportunity to express gratitude to God for opening for me this once-forbidden avenue to spiritual, physical, emotional and sexual healing.

The case examples and a broader sample of experiences described are compilations of my own experiences and those of the clients I have worked with as a "talking therapist" and a certified body worker. I draw from many years of experience as a social worker, involved in the prevention and treatment of child physical and sexual abuse. I have also been professionally trained in the art of body work and massage, having provided treatment to an array of clients. Although these case histories and examples are based on actual situations, in most instances the identifying details of these composites have been changed to protect individual privacy while maintaining the representative character of each description.

In addition, the material presented has been critiqued by a panel of professional therapists who are actively integrating body work with more traditional therapeutic traditions, theology and personal recovery paths. With their contribution and consultation, I am able to greatly increase the spectrum of clinical and personal experience, wisdom and client sample than I would otherwise have as a solitary practitioner.

Lastly, my insights, hunches and anecdotal experiences are corroborated by findings of scientific research and current theoretical exploration. In order to aid you in deciding for yourself, I cite from research and indicate my personal conclusions.

A word about the research is in order. I cite from research conducted on human beings, most often infants, as well as studies conducted on animals. Because of research guidelines, the research conducted on human infants is significantly more humane than that using animals. While I cite from animal research, I find it morally necessary to state that I do not support such activity. The suffering caused by animal research is immeasurable, since we often do to animals what we are unwilling to do to ourselves. I believe that ultimately the most significant findings come from human experiments, regardless of the participant.

My goal is to share my experience with you as encouragement in sorting out your beliefs about bodies in general, and your body in particular. My prayer is that you will explore the potential benefits of massage and body work and discover a similar source of spiritual communion between yourself and your God.

Carmen Renee Berry
December, 1993
Pasadena, California

INTRODUCTION

The impersonality of life in the Western world has become such that we have produced a race of untouchables.

Ashley Montagu

This is a book about bodies, your body and my body and the stories they have to tell. All too often, we treat our bodies as possessions that must be tamed into submission. Along with western medicine that "treats" bodies as sources of pathology, we view our own bodies with suspicion, if not contempt. Then we wonder why we lack clarity about our decisions, feel disappointed with our intimate relationships, and addictively medicate our fears and longings. Few of us listen to the stories our bodies are trying to tell.

This is also a book about touch, hurtful touch, healing touch, the lack of touch. Words like violent, cold, impersonal and technological describe how many of us experience the world today. Many of us feel more comfortable relating to each other via the safety of "distant" senses such as sight and hearing than by the senses that draw us close. Taste, smell, and most certainly touch, are by and large neglected, if not considered taboo.

This is also a book about trust. Safety is often sought, not in coming together and negotiating, but in dividing into special interest groups warring for supremacy. Violence in our streets escalates as more and more Americans hide guns under their pillows. Fear is rampant and blame is flung in every direction. Who can we trust? Where can we go for safety? What direction should we take to bring about the healing we so desperately need?

Our society is coming apart at the seams because we, as the individuals who comprise this society, are coming undone. Violence against the bodies of others comes more easily when we no longer honor our own bodies with respect. We don't know who to trust because we no longer trust ourselves. We have inherited an attitude toward our bodies that divides us from ourselves and from each other.

This book is for people who, like myself, have lost confidence in the directives given through traditional religious, political and medical institutions. Because of the crisis of trust, many have discarded western spirituality and medical practices for eastern approaches to grapple with these dilemmas. Unwilling to abandon my religious heritage, however, I have endeavored to reunite myself with my body from a western perspective. Consequently, I draw heavily on the support of western-based scientific research to support my belief that our bodies are trustworthy sources of guidance, information that can be discerned through touch.

Interest in approaching the body from new vantage points is rapidly growing. Alternative medical practices are being explored and discussed more openly. The body is becoming a legitimate subject among professional therapeutic and religious circles that previously shunned such conversation. A look around any book store today reveals a flood of new books on body-related subjects of health, massage, sexuality, and exercise. My hope and prayer is that my experience and ideas will contribute to this growing attempt to honor the body in a new way.

Part One
Your Body Never Lies

Chapter One

Your Body Never Lies

Anna, her knees locked tightly out of sight under the table, scooted the piece of lettuce once more across her plate.

"Are you OK?" Donna asked, eyeing the bedraggled lettuce. "You've hardly touched your lunch."

Leaning back with a huge sigh, Anna looked up at the ceiling and squinted her eyes as if watching a private scene too painful to describe. Glancing back at Donna, she said, "Oh, I'm fine. Just one of those days. No big deal, really."

"Then why aren't you eating? Is the salad bad?" Donna asked, turning her head and searching the room. "Maybe we should get the waiter back here and complain."

"No, please," Anna pleaded, sinking lower into her chair. "Don't embarrass me. The salad is fine, really."

"Then what?" Donna pushed. "You usually love this restaurant. I thought you'd enjoy doing something special. What is wrong?"

"I've lost my appetite, that's all. It's nothing really. Please, can we just drop this and talk about something else? Anything else?" Anna jabbed at the piece of lettuce, this time skewering it.

"Sure," Donna said, leaning back, crossing her arms. "Talk about anything you'd like, but don't expect me to believe you. I know you, Anna, and you're keeping something from me. It's written all over you."

◆ ◆ ◆ ◆

Adam rubbed the back of his neck as he reread the memo under the dim lamp on his desk. Except for this one light, the office was dark. His coworkers had long since gone home for the evening. Adam had intended to leave with them, until the memo from his supervisor appeared on his desk.

"Nothing I do is good enough for this guy. He's a real pain in the neck," Adam muttered to himself. Without looking, his right hand searched an open desk drawer for the bottle of pain killers. Having popped three tablets into his mouth, Adam rubbed his temples briefly and thought, "Well, I might as well call Sue. I won't be able to make it home for dinner. This will take me all night."

Reaching for the phone, he thought angrily, "I could work so much faster if it weren't for this headache! Why do I always get these migraines when the pressure is on and I need to concentrate most?"

◆ ◆ ◆ ◆

"Phil? Phil? Is that you?" Andrea called after the man who had quickly passed her in the store aisle.

Turning, first with a look of confusion then delighted recognition, Phil beamed. "Andrea! I walked right past you!"

Grinning back, Andrea teased, "I thought that was you. Still wearing the suit I gave you for Christmas a couple years back, huh?"

Glancing down briefly, Phil nodded, "Not much has changed with me, but you!" Phil leaned back and gave her the once over. "You look great, uh, different somehow."

Twirling around once, Andrea giggled, "I'm walking on air these days! So much has happened since we broke up, some wonderful things actually."

"Well, it shows!" Phil smiled. "You glow from your head to your feet!"

Reading Your Body's Map

We may say we feel fine, but the knot in our stomachs reveal our anxiety or confusion. Our neck muscles twist and tighten, leading to pounding headaches that alert us to dangerous levels of stress or unexpressed rage. When we are happy, our bodies celebrate with excited energy, aligned body posture, and a healthy glow on our skin that others can see. Like a road map, our bodies reflect the terrain of our emotions, indicate historical points of interest, and show us how to reach our desired destination of wholeness and healing.

Through a variety of conditions including muscle tension, skin resilience, depth of breath, skeletal structure or brain size, our bodies reveal our past experience and reflect how we genuinely feel. No matter what covering we may put over our bodies, we cannot erase the personalized and accurate record we carry within our bodies. If we know how to read our body "map" (and if we heed the directions as well), we can proceed down life's highway confident of our direction.

Unfortunately many of us do not know how to read our body maps well enough to gain needed guidance. Many are confused about who we are and how we feel. Far too many of us are lost.

Misreading Your Body Map

Sitting on the edge of my chair, I enthusiastically described to my counselor my most recent insight. Being a therapist myself, I was able to apply my psychological training to my own life, coming up with a variety of elaborate explanations for my feelings and self-abusive behaviors. Each week, more insight. Each week, minimal change.

Fortunately my therapist was unwilling to allow my brilliant observations to obscure the fact that I was making little progress.

Propelled by adrenaline, I was still "forgetting" to eat, sometimes dropping as many as ten pounds in a week. My sleep was often disrupted by terrifying nightmares, jarring me awake. Work consumed my waking hours, leaving little opportunity for intimacy or relaxation. Frightening, but obscure images skirted around the edges of consciousness. I talked on and on but not much changed.

"Carmen," my therapist confronted me one afternoon (after a particularly insightful comment on my part, I might add), "you are living in your head. And nothing is really going to change until you get into your body."

I looked down at my body in bewilderment. "My body? What does my body have to do with anything?"

"Exactly my point," she smiled.

My body map revealed it all, but the message was lost on me. I misread my body map in three ways: I disregarded my body, I neglected my body, and I rejected my body.

I Disregarded My Body

As I drove down a familiar stretch of the freeway late one night, my thoughts were on the day's events. Suddenly the tail lights of the car in front of me beamed bright red. Abruptly emerging from my haze, I saw the blue and red flashing lights atop a fire truck and a police car. An accident! Sizzling flares lined the roadside, directing us to form a single file lane around the tangled cars. Without these signs warning of danger on the road, I could have unwittingly crashed into the disabled vehicles, adding my car to the wreckage.

Similarly, our bodies warn us about impending danger. When our bodies' sense potential harm, the lights flash and the flares go off: our palms sweat, the heart beats faster, our breath rate increases. If we read these signs accurately and respond by protecting ourselves, we avoid unnecessary damage. However, if we ignore these signals, we suffer.

I hate to admit that I learned to accurately interpret roadside warnings long before I was adept at reading my body's danger signals. Simply stated, I disregarded my body map because I didn't believe my body had anything important to reveal. I was concerned solely with academic and career achievement, viewing my body as a machine that carried my brain from library to classroom to workplace. Disdain for my body was reinforced by a religious upbringing that declared the "flesh" as evil and untrustworthy.

Lacking self-awareness, I failed to have a sense of where I began or ended. Unable to delineate physical or emotional boundaries, my attempts to relate to others often resulted in pain rather than nurture. Repeatedly suffering from destructive relationships, I ignored the queasiness of my stomach each time I was in the presence of people who meant me harm. I medicated the dizzy pain of migraines rather than recognizing the dangerous levels of stress in my life. Sleeping pills became my response to insomnia rather than questioning the source of my agitation. I ignored the signs my body offered and as a result, I suffered.

When I treated my body with disrespect, I unknowingly treated other people's bodies disrespectfully as well. This, of course, undermined my attempts at intimacy. Who wanted to be intimate with someone who resented touch, closeness, and affection? Believe me, not many. Even though I felt desperate at times for love and affection, my self-inflicted hatred of my own body barred me from getting what I needed.

I was afraid to get close, afraid I'd be touched in scary ways. Scarier still was the fear of never being touched at all. Like so many who disregard their bodies, I swung from one extreme to the other; I succumbed to bouts of neediness by using touch in inappropriate ways, then pushed away all forms of physical nurture, which left me trapped in isolation.

As I look around, I see that I am not alone in this malady. Many of us do not navigate touch in a self-respectful, nurturing way. Rather, it is common to eroticize our need for touch: we use, misuse and over-use sex as a primary means for nurturance. Some become promiscuous, even addicted to sexual contact. Others become "touch avoidant" and push away all nurturing touch. When we lock the body away in the dungeon of our disdain, sexuality is often a fellow prisoner. Our bodies suffer, our relationships suffer as we misread our body maps and take detour after detour.

I Neglected My Body

I neglected my body's legitimate needs in a variety of ways: I grabbed meals on the run, sacrificing good nutrition for expedience. Sleep was a luxury that was sacrificed regularly to meet work deadlines. I tended to medicate illnesses to silence my body, rather than address the underlying source of my pain.

Since intellectual exercise was the only workout I felt had merit, it was hard for me to justify physical exercise. One afternoon when I was still in college, I was studying on the lawn in front of the library. A friend jogged up, puffing after a workout. Looking at her with disgust, I asked, "How can you waste valuable work time on jumping around?" She laughed, thinking I was joking and jogged off.

Watching her as she ran down the street, I thought to myself, "Perhaps exercise could help me study longer." But since I wasn't inclined to exert myself physically anyway, I dismissed that idea and returned to my books. Viewing my body as having something important to teach me was inconceivable. Like too many others I've met, my body was to be my servant, not my teacher.

As a consequence of this neglect, my health began to suffer. Instead of enjoying the energy of a healthy body, a daily adrenaline rush of anxiety propelled me through the day. Rather than honoring my body's need for rest, I relied on migraine headaches and menstrual cramps as excuses to take a day off. My overall health and vitality declined as my weakened immune system was unable to combat even the mildest of viruses. By the time I was through graduate school and into the work force, it was common for me to miss as much as a week of work a month to some physical ailment.

I Rejected My Body

Since I believed that the important things in life took place in my mind, anything about myself that was "nonintellectual" was rejected. Artificial battle lines were drawn between my "head" and my "heart," between my thoughts and my feelings. I was especially embarrassed by emotions, those wild, unruly sensations that seemed to defy logic or control. In those days, if someone asked me how I felt, I told them what I thought.

Foolishly, I believed I could control my feelings by ignoring them, hiding them or pretending they just didn't exist at all. But feelings do not evaporate simply because they are unwelcome. Rather, emotions that are not allowed authentic expression can be stored in the body evidenced by an achy shoulder, repetitive clenching of the toes, or an overwhelming sense of fatigue. Like a beach ball pushed underwater, popping up in unexpected places, my emotions found a home in my body and erupted in unpredictable and often distressing ways. Living purely out of my head gave my rejected emotions more potency, not less, as my muscles knotted with tension, my breathing grew sluggish, my immune system grew more deficient in fighting off the mildest infections, and waves of unexplained feelings grew more powerful. I remember sitting at my desk one afternoon for hours, staring at the wall, weighed down with depression and hopelessness, trying to "think" myself back into productivity. It didn't work.

Since I was more adept at expressing my ideas than my feelings, my relationships with others suffered. Putting words to feelings was difficult and most certainly uncomfortable. My conversations with friends tended to focus solely on intellectual pursuits—what we had read, what we were doing professionally, what we thought. Expressing love and intimacy scared me because doing so put me into contact with a body from which I was estranged.

Looking back, I can see time and again, when heeding my body map could have saved me time, energy, and a great deal of needless suffering. This suffering originated in a commonly held misconception. Like others, I perceived my "self" as separate from my body. James Nelson, noted author, points out that it is easier for us to "speak of the 'personality' as identical with the self than it is to speak of the body and the self as one. 'I am a personality' simply sounds more natural than 'I am a body.' "[1]

I did not experience myself as a body, rather I *had* a body and we were at war. "It" against me, my body was an unruly slave that only got my attention when the news was bad—a lingering sinus infection, a throbbing broken toe, a frightening chest pain, a sore neck muscle, a cancer scare, another sleepless night.

I didn't realize that my body and I were on the same team. We *were.* the same team. The only difference between us was that I knew how to lie. My body always told the truth.

Benefits of Following Our Body Maps

On my therapist's recommendation, I agreed to meet with a body worker for a few sessions to see what might be learned. Skeptical, if not a true "unbeliever," I made my first appointment. On the drive over I promised myself, "If I'm not comfortable with this new experience, I'll say so and leave. And I'll only have a second session if I feel safe." I then proceeded to imagine the many reasons I would give to my counselor for why this body work deal was bogus, unintellectual, and "fringy" at best.

Starting slowly, moving at my pace, the body worker created an atmosphere of safety and concern. Noticing my nervousness, she told me that I was in control of the session, and that she would follow my lead. More comfortable with words than silence, I began talking about what I thought about my body. Kindly, she instructed me to listen in silence for what my body may say. The silence was agitating for me at first, as I was unaccustomed to communicating in a nonverbal channel. But I waited. I listened. And soon my body revealed accurate information about myself, truth that I had been able to deny intellectually. Sore knots in my back revealed anger I didn't want to acknowledge. Shortness of breath uncovered anxiety I wanted to hide. Tears flowed as my calf muscles were gently massaged, giving me a long needed opportunity to grieve. That first session lasted no more than an hour, but the impact will be with me for a lifetime. I took the first step toward understanding that my body actually contains wisdom and that, through accurately reading my body map, that wisdom can be mine.

Your body map can be understood through a variety of body-oriented activities and therapies. For example, one friend of mine best understands herself through movement. While dancing to music, she uncovers emotions such as anger, fear, love, contentment, or longing. Movement gives her the opportunity to first identify and then express these emotions. In addition, by the end of a dance, she often has clarity and insight about a particularly niggling problem. As she accurately reads her body map through movement, she gains guidance and a sense of confidence about future decisions.

Another friend gains guidance from her body through breathing awareness. She often stops in conversation to monitor her breath and discern what her breath reveals about what she's feeling. When she is frightened or angry, she often calms herself through deepening her breath. She has even remembered long-forgotten experiences by either exaggerating her breath or purposefully slowing her breath down.

These are but two of the ways the body can provide wisdom to you. I have benefitted from these methods, but the most powerful for me, by far, has been through the avenue of touch. I have become a willing student, enjoying the many benefits of reading my body map through massage and body work. These benefits include increased enjoyment of intimacy, an increase in health and vitality, and an integration of the past with the present.

Increased Enjoyment of Intimacy

One of the first benefits I received from massage was the discovery that I had legs and feet! Certainly, whenever I stubbed my toes or skinned my knee, I was painfully aware of my lower limbs. But on a daily basis, I was completely unaware of the bottom half of my body.

The experience of body work has helped me locate the boundaries of my body and to fill out my body so that I now am able to inhabit all of myself. At points I have resisted knowing the extent of my body because I felt ashamed about the shape, size, or firmness of various body parts. In an effort to feel good about myself, I disowned those parts that I disliked. However, healing of my low self image came through the opposite course of action. The more completely I have experienced my body and acknowledged all parts of myself, the better I have come to feel about my body as well.

My experience is common. In fact, research affirms the assertion that an accurate sense of one's body is the basis for healthy self esteem. Dr. Sandra Weiss, a nurse and researcher on infancy, conducted a study of children ages eight through ten to assess how their touch experiences helped or hindered their awareness of their bodies. Her research team found that the children with the highest regard for their bodies were those who had the highest awareness of their bodies. This body awareness was gained through nurturing, stimulating touch received by their parents. Positive touch had three components: 1) touch was experienced by the child as comfortable, 2) touch occurred over a large extent of the child's body, and 3) touch was intense enough to gain the child's attention.[2]

It is not too late to develop an accurate sense of boundaries and repair a poor body image. Massage and body work can provide the kind of touch we need to experience ourselves fully. As is true for young children, healing touch needs to be comfortable, involve a large extent of your body and be intense and engaging enough to gain your attention. Massage and body work offer a unique opportunity for this special kind of touch, and can go a long way to repair the deficits of the past.

Unfortunately, most people I talk to tell me they do not receive the amount or kind of touch they need. Most of our social interactions consist of verbal exchange, even though, as touch researcher Saul Schanberg from Duke University asserts, "Touch is ten times stronger than verbal or visual contact."[3] We need to touch and be touched, and yet few of us enjoy the physical interchange we desperately need. If we do touch others, most often touch is reserved solely for the sexual arena.

While sexual touch can, indeed, be nurturing and satisfying, deriving all of our touch nurturance from sex can leave even the most sexually active adult longing for other kinds of nurturing touch. Some, driven by the need for touch, engage in sex more often than actually desired, since sex seems to be the only "legitimate" way in this society to share the experience of touch. Massage and body work can provide you with safe, nurturing, nonsexual touch experiences that nourish your skin, give a more accurate sense of body boundaries, and satisfy your emotional longings for intimacy.

As a consequence of receiving the touch we need, our intimate relationships can be enhanced. First, we are less likely to place excessive demands on our sexual experiences. Instead, we are free to enjoy physical intimacy with realistic expectations.

Secondly, nurturing touch helps us gain a greater sense of body awareness. As we become more aware of our body boundaries, we are more able to protect ourselves from harmful interactions with others. An army must know the geographical boundaries of a territory in order to station guards at selected outposts. Similarly, we need to know where to draw the line between ourselves and those who might hurt us. Accurate body awareness is the foundation of self-protection.

Thirdly, as our self-protection skills increase, so does our sense of safety. The safer we feel, the closer we can draw to those we love and who want to love us back. Our bodies signal us of danger or safety, through the feeling in the pit of our stomachs, the amount and temperature of moisture on our palms, or level of stress in our jaws. By accurately reading our body maps and then acting on this information, we can better avoid hurtful relationships and invest wisely in nurturing intimacy.

Touch between ourselves and loved ones becomes more nurturing as we learn to trust and enjoy nurturing touch from our body workers. I have become a more physically affectionate person due to massage and body work. Affectionate touch shared between lovers, family, or friends can be expressed more freely and enjoyed more fully.

Increase in Health and Vitality

Our fast-paced and high-pressure society pushes most of us toward excessive work and overcommitment. When stressed, a number of hormones are released into our bodies. In small quantities or for short periods of time, these hormones help increase awareness and capacity to respond to potential danger. If, however, stress is a way of life, rather than experienced as periodic episodes, these hormones cease to be helpful.

Instead, the steady flow of hormones, especially adrenalin, creates what Archibald Hart, in his book, The Hidden Link Between Adrenalin and Stress, refers to as "stress disease." Hart writes, "In addition to coronary and artery disease, many other kinds and symptoms of stress damage can be traced back to the excessive flow of adrenalin: headaches (tension and migraine), gastric problems, ulcers, and high blood pressure."[4] Medical research has amply illustrated that stress diminishes the body's ability to fight disease. Stress takes its toll slowly, through sapping our bodies' capacity to effectively ward off illness. An impaired immune system opens the body to a myriad of painful, even life-threatening diseases.

In addition, some diseases are known to be caused by the disruption of normal functioning traced directly back to an increase of stress. Anyone suffering from a stomach ulcer knows the discomfort caused by acid secreted into the stomach. The excessive flow of acid, triggered by bouts of stress, can actually damage tissue and decrease the stomach's ability to effectively digest food, needed for overall health and vitality.[5]

Living in the fast lane, driven by the many demands of daily life, can drown out our bodies' attempts to get our attention. Rather than accurately read our bodies' loud, and often physically painful messages, we may try to medicate our bodies into silence. A. Hart points out that "all of this can lead to an increase in the use of alcohol, cigarettes, and drugs. And these, in turn, can take their toll by causing further illnesses and damage in and of themselves."[6]

Massage and body work give us opportunity to STOP. Stop the running, stop the intensity, stop the dangerous flow of adrenalin. Massage assists in managing the stressful demands of daily living through a variety of health enhancing experiences:

- deepening the breath, drawing more oxygen into the blood stream
- releasing of knots of tension stored in muscles throughout the body
- decreasing heart rate and blood pressure
- redistributing blood throughout the body for proper cell nourishment and waste removal.

While not a guaranteed way to avoid all physical maladies, I believe regular massage can decrease the chances of stress-related illness. In addition, massage can help us become acquainted with our bodies so that, should we contract an illness, we will be more able to recognize the changes in our bodies and the specific symptoms of disease. When I relax on the massage table, I am more able to recognize the signs my body map offers and then respond in a healing manner.

Integration of the Past with the Present

Parked by the side of the road, I studied the road map and chewed my lip in indecision. This area was unfamiliar to me and I had gotten turned around. I looked down one street searching for some familiar feature.

"Hmmm," I questioned myself, "have I gone down that road before?" Looking in a different direction, I continued, "or did I come up that way?" What a dilemma. Until I could figure out which direction I had come from, I wouldn't be able to locate where I was now on the map. And until I knew where I was, I wouldn't be able to get to the place I wanted to go.

Life's experiences are similar. To get to where we want to go, we need to know where we are and where we've been. Effective travel, across town or through life, is dependent upon our ability to integrate the past, present, and our future destination.

Unfortunately, many people have an obscure recollection of the past. In fact, some adults are unable to remember certain experiences, large sections of their childhood, or even their childhoods in entirety. The inability to tell one's story, accurately and completely, significantly diminishes the capacity for creating a life in the present that is satisfying, stable, and safe.

"Forgotten" memories are often remembered in the recesses of our unconscious minds and in our bodies. Since God designed us as beings who long for truth and unity, all parts of ourselves struggle toward wholeness. Our hidden secrets strain against the chains and cry out to us for freedom. If we are quiet, sometimes we can hear these cries, which come to us in many forms.

For example, we may become overwhelmed by strong emotion that seems to appear out of nowhere. Or we may feel nothing at all.

Our bodies may curl forward, unable to stand straight, to illustrate our inner agony. Or our back muscles may become as tight as metal rods in rigid defiance and rage. Our toes may frantically grip at the ground, fearful of relaxing and "flying off" the planet. Unexplained fears and phobias may deter daily functioning. Certain colors may frighten us, specific smells distress us, and people with particular characteristics can cause us to catch our breath. Our bodies remember and try to tell us truth. Body work is an extremely effective method for discerning this truth, especially those aspects that seem most difficult to consciously retain. To be whole, we must accurately read our body maps and honestly acknowledge where we have been. Only then can we truly know who we are right now and how to move into the future with confidence.

Reading Our Body Maps

The more adept I have become at reading my body map, the more accurately I am able to interpret my body's guidance. The more I act on this wisdom, the more change I enjoy, real change, flesh-and-blood change.

The touch I receive from massage and body work helps me pay closer attention to my body. I take the experiences to my "talking" therapist, who then helps me put my experiences into words. In tandem, body work and talking therapy have broken through my intellectual head games and brought healing down into my body, into my psyche, into my soul, into myself.

As a consequence, my anxiety attacks have grown less intense and occur less often. Feelings once trapped beneath the mask of my depression are more fully expressed and enjoyed. Through regular sessions, my muscles release the stress and tension accumulated through a fast-paced lifestyle. Haunting mysteries of past traumatic experience are coming clear, finally giving me the opportunity to put those old ghosts to rest.

I am still on a journey of healing and growth. My problems were not solved overnight, but the positive changes I now enjoy in all areas of my life have been possible because of the healing that has taken place and continues to take place between me and my body.

I was so impressed with the changes in my own life that, five years after my introduction to body work, I received training to become a body worker myself. In the past several years, I have worked with many clients who also have benefited from believing their bodies and receiving the healing power of touch. I now travel across the country leading workshops for those who are open to learning from the wisdom of the body.

I believe that body work can facilitate a more stress-free, healthy life in the present, as well as be a powerful healing agent of wounds and memories of the past. Milton Trager, the founder of Tragerwork®, a form of body work, says, "Every shimmer of tissue is sending a message to the unconscious mind in the form of a positive feeling experience. It is the accumulation of these positive patterns that can offset the negative patterns to where the positive can take over."[7]

What can your body map reveal to you? What do the knots in your shoulders mean? When your lower back aches, what message are you being sent? Are the secrets of your childhood buried in your breathing pattern, the tension in your left thigh, your pounding headache? How can honoring your body strengthen your relationship with God? These are some of the questions we will be exploring in the following chapters. I invite you to join me in a special adventure of unlocking the mysteries of healing and love recorded within the uniqueness of your body map.

<hr>

NOTES

1 James B. Nelson. Embodiment: An Approach to Sexuality and Christian Theology (Minneapolis: Augsburg, 1978), 38.

2 Sandra J. Weiss. "Parental Touch and the Child's Body Image," in The Many Facets of Touch, ed. Catherine Caldwell Brown (New Jersey: Johnson & Johnson Baby Products Company, 1984), 133.

3 Saul Schanberg, Quote from interview with author, November 22, 1993.

4 Archibald Hart. The Hidden Link between Adrenalin and Stress: The Exciting New Breakthrough That Helps You Overcome Stress Damage. (Waco, TX: Word, 1986), 12.

5 Hart, 7.

6 Ibid. 7.

7 Richard Leviton. "Moving with Milton Trager," East West Magazine, January 1988, 57, 58.

Chapter Two

Too Young To Remember?

Jake held his eight-month old son tightly in his arms, grateful the doctor had said Teddy would be fine. "Certainly took a nasty bump," the emergency room physician commented. Jake swallowed tears as he recalled how he had watched, helpless and in horror, as the car had careened out of control on the ice and ran into a tree. Rushed to the hospital, both he and his son were shaken up. They each had a couple of scrapes but were otherwise unharmed.

Giving Jake a smile of reassurance, the doctor said, "It'll take a little time for the bruises to heal, but he'll be fine."

Jake sighed with relief, "Thanks, Doctor. At least he's too young to remember this."

◆ ◆ ◆ ◆

Were you ever too young to remember? Does the body remember the past? If so, how much? What can your body really tell you about yourself and your many life experiences?

I believe that we have underestimated infants' ability to understand and record their experiences. Because adults are unable to converse with infants, we have had the tendency to conclude that infants are unaware of what goes on around them. We've tended to believe that babies somehow "forget" experiences that occur during infancy.

Some cognitive theorists, for example, place a higher value on verbal skills than other forms of communication such as touch or eye contact.[1] Some have assumed that if infants could not communicate verbally, then they were unable to communicate at all. In fact, some theorists believe that an infant is unable to even feel what he or she cannot verbalize. As one clinician told me, "We don't seem to give credit to any living creature that doesn't talk."[2] As a consequence of this theoretical blind spot, much that occurs to us as infants, especially in the early months of life, has been minimized or even disregarded.

Even though some branches of psychological inquiry, most notably psychoanalysis, have stressed the importance of early childhood experiences in our psychological development and adult functioning, many theorists, parent educators, and health professionals have sorely underestimated how complicated and competent we are from birth. In fact, initial life experiences, especially those involving touch, can have a significant impact on the rest of our lives.

Our ability to relate well with ourselves and others later in life is rooted in our early experiences as infants. We have not known, until recently, just how important these early experiences can be. In fact, much of what we now know about early infancy and subsequent adult functioning comes from studies conducted in the past forty, perhaps most importantly, the past twenty years. Since it takes time for scientific findings to become part of everyday practices, most of us were raised by parents influenced by thinkers who speculated about infancy without the assistance of this research.

Researchers are discovering that, as infants, we are much more aware, much more capable of understanding and organizing information, and much more impacted by experiences, especially touch, than previously suspected. We are learning that by the time you and I are able to talk, much of our fundamental cognitive and emotional mapping has already been established. Infants are born with a variety of innate abilities and the capacity to organize information that reaches back into the womb. In fact, *we are never too young to remember.* We even remember experiences prior to our birth.

To better understand our bodies, we must travel back, not merely to childhood experiences but to the time prior to our births when we were aquatic mammals floating in the nurturing sea of the womb.

In the Womb

When you and I were around an inch long, some six weeks after conception in our mothers' wombs, we had no eyes by which to see or ears by which to hear. We did, however, have one way to experience ourselves or the world around us—through our skin.[3]

As a developing organism in the womb, our skin provided us with our *very first sensations.* Our skin gave us initial information about who we might be and where on earth we might be floating. Caressed gently by the soft folds of our mothers' wombs, feeling the stroking ripples of the amniotic fluid as our mothers moved, our little bodies received the ultimate massage.

In the womb, the skin and the central nervous system are linked, originating from the same tissue. Dr. Ashley Montagu, author of Touching, writes, "The nervous system is . . . a buried part of the skin, or alternatively the skin may be regarded as an exposed portion of the nervous system. It would, therefore, improve our understanding of these matters if we were to think and speak of the skin as the external nervous system . . . "[4]

The brain develops using information gathered through the nervous system, especially the skin. The skin picks up information about the outside world and sends it to the brain for processing. The amount and type of stimulation the skin receives impacts not only the information the brain stores but also how well the brain is able to process and store that information.

Perhaps one way to understand this process is to imagine the brain to be like a computer. Suppose you had a computer that had a small capacity to store information. However, the more you touched the keys and put information into the computer, you found that the storage capacity actually got larger. If the computer was not used, then the capacity remained small.

The brain develops in a similar way. The more the brain is stimulated, the better it functions, the larger it grows, and the more efficiently it processes information. The more the skin is stimulated, the more the brain is stimulated. Therefore, the touch we receive, from conception on, impacts the development of our brains.

As the brain tissue develops, a "cognitive map" or structure of cells form in the brain tissue through repeated sensory stimulation. Sandra J. Weiss, in "Parental Touch and the Child's Body Image," writes:

> A cell assemblage or map may be described as a cortical representation that is formed through frequently repeated sensory stimulations and neuromuscular excitations of the body. In this way, each separate tactile [or touch] experience becomes related to the next and is ordered cognitively. The implications of such a process are that initially developed [brain] representations may affect the core experiences and resulting meanings that an individual comes to understand.[5]

Touch experiences, even before you were born, helped to influence how well your brain functions and stores information. Every time your mother moved, your tiny body received an all-encompassing massage. Every day, every hour the sides of your mother's womb stroked and caressed your body from head to toe. This touch stimulated your skin, which in turn influenced the development of your mental map, the patterning of your mind.

Now that we have moved from that solitary, aquatic massage chamber of the womb to an atmospheric and often stressful social environment, the skin, as well as other sensory organs, continue to play a vital role in our development and life satisfaction. We are born with five senses: the sense of taste, smell, sight, hearing and touch. Each of these senses has corresponding sensory organs: tongue, nose, eyes, ears, and skin. While all five senses are important for a complete experience of the world around us, I believe our most important sensory organ is the skin. In addition to be being the largest organ in our body, the skin has a massive representation in the brain itself.[6]

We may underestimate the vital necessity of our skin. Many of us view our outer covering as something to tan in the summer, to cover with creams each night to ward off wrinkling, or to wrap up in sweaters on a brisk winter night. Our skin and the skin of a loved one may take on special interest when we contemplate a romantic, erotic encounter. Skin is often seen merely as packaging used in the effort to market ourselves in a critical, weight-conscious, "hard body" society.

Many of us regard our bodies, and especially the skin, as secondary to the emotional, intellectual, relational, or spiritual aspects of life. Certainly traditional psychotherapy, recovery approaches, and many religions have made no special effort to address the needs of the body as a whole or the particular needs of the skin. It is easy to overlook our bodies, and specifically our skin, unless something goes awry and we are confronted with discomfort, pain, or disease.

Our First Experiences Following Birth

Even though Carmella's eyelids were heavy and she ached from the long labor, she longed to hold her newborn son. As if reading her mind, Jeff, her husband, appeared in the doorway with Sammy in his arms.

"Ooooo, my little Sammy," Carmella beamed as his little body relaxed against her tummy. "Are you hungry for your first meal from Mommy?" Moving her son to her breast, Sammy was soon lunching away with vigor.

Jeff grinned, "His first meal and he's already a pro!"

◆ ◆ ◆ ◆

As a newborn, you had the opportunity to experience every aspect of life for the *very first time.* One by one, specific memories were collected, initially recorded as isolated and unrelated events.

We experience each of these events as participants, not merely as casual observers watching television. Every physical event or experience has a corresponding emotional response experienced in the body. As you were cuddled and nursed, your muscles relaxed, your breath became slow and steady and you felt safe and loved. When your diapers were wet, your muscles tightened, you gasped air as you cried, and you felt distress and discomfort. Each experience evoked feelings, new feelings, odd feelings, fun feelings, scary feelings—all of which were experienced in your body. Emotions, as well as the experiences that triggered those feelings, are stored in the body's memory.

While our bodies remember past experiences, I do not believe each event is remembered equally. While initially each experience was remembered as an independent event, eventually separate, day-to-day events were no longer stored as separate memories. Rather, they were collapsed into memories of *patterns.* These memories of patterns served to shape how our bodies responded to the world around us on a regular basis, patterns we may now take for granted. For example, the first time we felt hungry, we cried, not knowing what to expect. We were fed. The next time we cried, there was a memory of our first feeding and a blossoming hope that we might be fed again. As we were cuddled and nursed, our muscles relaxed and our shape conformed to the contours of our caretaker's body. Lips sucked nourishment into our stomachs as our digestive and elimination systems were stimulated. Feelings of satisfaction and safety became familiar. We became aware, not merely of this particular feeding but of the patterned experience of "being fed." And "being fed" was more than an intellectual concept; it was a body-based and emotionally-laden experience in which we fully participated.

Babies are born with the innate ability to detect patterns among experiences and feelings. Our brains begin to notice similarities among experiences: the enjoyment of this fragrance seems similar to the smell enjoyed previously, this wet diaper stings the skin much like the last damp diaper, this mouthful of warm, sweet milk tastes quite like our last meal. Dr. Daniel Stern, noted researcher and Professor of Psychiatry at Cornell University Medical Center, explains:

> By the time the baby has registered the second or third similar specific memory, his mind will start to operate on those two recalled affective experiences and will do the things that we now expect human minds to do beginning from very early on in life. They will identify patterns to try to see what was the same in each of those recalled experiences [memories]. That is, they will search for the features that are common to each memory.[7]

As each single event was layered onto the next single event, our bodies recognized a pattern of feeling hungry, crying for food, and being fed. Our bodies stored the sequential wisdom of "being fed." We began to respond in similar ways each time we felt hungry until our muscles, skin, bones, and breath set down the foundation for our own personal body map. Likewise, our soiled diapers engaged our full attention by annoying our skin and upsetting our mood. After alerting those around us with a hearty cry (thereby utilizing our bodies as an avenue of self-care), we welcomed a clean bottom and a fresh, dry diaper. If we were nurtured on a regular basis, our bodies learned to anticipate living in safety.[8]

Remembering Trauma

"Will you please check Bennie and see why he's crying?" Kitty asked Ally, her teenage daughter as Kitty headed the car up the freeway on-ramp. "He's crying like there's something really wrong!"

Reaching around the car seat that held her boisterous brother, Ally said, "Oh, he's got a little blister on his leg!" Unsnapping the seat belt, she lifted Bennie into her arms. "Is that better, Bennie?" she cooed. From the back seat Ally reported, "Looks like the sun heated up the metal bracket on the car seat and it burned his skin. No wonder he was putting up a fuss!"

◆ ◆ ◆ ◆

As infants like Bennie, we responded to pain on a variety of levels. Our muscles may have tightened, the heart rate may have sped up, our voices may have been called upon to make our distress known to those around us who could help us. We did what we could to protect ourselves from experiencing more pain.

If all of our experiences were positive, we'd have little need to protect ourselves from harm. Unfortunately, many difficult and threatening events come our way over the course of a lifetime, events that our bodies work hard to anticipate, avoid, or overcome.

To anticipate and avoid future trauma, our bodies remember events that are out of the ordinary, traumatic, or odd. Memories of traumatic experiences are stored with "emotion-linked chemicals in the body and the brain. When a childhood trauma occurs, the child is in a highly emotionally charged state, causing certain hormones known as neuropeptides or 'messenger molecules' to be released into the body when the memory is being stored."[9]

Traumatic experiences may be irregular occurrences in an otherwise routine and safe existence. We all have had our share of falling off our bicycles and skinning our knees or underestimating how hot a pan might be and burning our fingers. Children are curious, not always aware of the dangers of exploration, and painfully discover just how high, how hot, or how hard something might be. The more unusual these accidents were for you, the more likely you are to remember.

Sadly, some traumatic events are not accidental. Too many children in our society are traumatized through the intentional misuse or neglect perpetrated by their caretakers. All forms of child abuse are traumatic and harmful to the child's body. Dr. Gail Goodman, a psychologist at the State University of New York, Buffalo, writes, "Child abuse involves actions directed against a child's body. The violation of trivial expectations would probably not be very memorable. The violation of one's body is." [10]

Many who are abused as children are rarely abused *on solely one occasion.* Rather, abuse victims experience a *pattern of abuse* in their childhoods that may continue, in some form or another, into adulthood. In much the same way that the body remembers patterns of positive experiences, such as feeding or regular diaper changes, the body also records patterns of trauma and abuse.

If our needs were repetitively ignored, we came to distrust those around us. Our muscles may have routinely tightened to protect ourselves. Our shoulders may have hunched, our toes may have clenched, our jaws may have locked. If we repetitively held our breath in fear or anxiety, the muscles around our lungs may have developed shallow breathing patterns. If our arms were pushed away when we reached out for an embrace, we may have stopped trying. Instead, our arms may have learned to push away a comforting touch. These repetitive responses to pain, discomfort, or rejection often become ingrained in our bodies.

Without knowing it, we may now use this ingrained response whenever we feel afraid. Since this routine was established at an early age, we may not even be aware of what our bodies are doing;

we have grown accustomed to the ritualized response. In their book, Embodying Healing, psychologist Robert Timms and certified massage therapist, Patrick Connors, write "The body and the mind together then enact some kind of escape or avoidance routine that may become nearly automatic and may require a large expenditure of time and physical or emotional resources."[11]

Often we think of memory as a task for our brains alone. However, it is critical to recognize that our bodies, as a whole, record and respond to patterns of experience. In addition to our mental responses, our bodies rally in self-protection through the rate of your heartbeat, the rhythm of your breath, the sweat on your palms, the glance of your eyes, the tightness of your stomach, and the quickness of your thoughts. In fact, every experience you've had involved body sensations that can be anchored in the tissue itself.

I believe that God designed our bodies to record our experiences in an organized fashion. Each touch, each response, each moment contributes to the development of our body map. Patterns of experiences are noted. Odd, new, or variant events are remembered. From conception, you were able to learn from your experiences and then to remember that learning, taking the memory from one moment into the next.

Just as we use a map to find our way around a new, exciting city, we can also learn to read our bodies' symbols to better understand what forces have shaped us. Our body maps are reliable sources of information.

Our challenge is to accurately interpret the body's special map. If time is taken to properly understand the personal way each body structures and stores information, amazing wisdom can be gleaned. We can be pointed to experiences of deficit or abuse, perhaps no longer available to our conscious minds. Our bodies may speak of our need for nurturance or healing. Through prayerful consideration of what our bodies tell us, we can determine which direction will provide the best opportunities for meeting our needs.

Notes

1 Constance Maria Lillas, "Alexithymia: Etiology and Treatment Implications for Psychoanalysis," (Ph.D. diss., Newport Psychoanalytic Institute, 1992), 48.

2 Constance Maria Lillas, Quote from interview with author, December 1992.

3 Ashley Montagu, Touching: The Human Significance of Skin, Third Edition (New York: Harper & Row, 1986), 4.

4 Ibid.

5 Sandra Weiss, "Parental Touch and the Child's Body Image," in The Many Facets of Touch, ed. Catherine Caldwell Brown (New Jersey: Johnson & Johnson Baby Products Company, 1984), 131.

6 Montagu, Touching, 14.

7 Daniel N. Stern, "Affect in the Context of the Infant's Lived Experience: Some Considerations" International Journal of Psycho-Analysis v.69 (1988): 233.

8 Ibid. 233-34.

9 Robert Timms and Patrick Connors, Embodying Healing: Integrating Bodywork and Psychotherapy in Recovery from Childhood Sexual Abuse (Orwell: The Safer Society Press, 1992), 31.

10 Gail S. Goodman, Quoted in Heidi Vanderbilt, "Incest: A Chilling Report," Lear's Magazine, February 1992, 57.

11 Timms and Connors, Embodying Healing, 24.

Part Two
Your Body Remembers

Chapter Three

Your Body Remembers
Attentive Touch

Pamela had just set down the receiver when the phone rang again. A wave of fatigue and emptiness swept over her as she lifted the receiver to her ear.

"Hello?" she asked wearily, thinking to herself, "Who could this be? Who else needs me?"

"Pam?" the caller asked, "It's Zach. Got a minute? I'm in a jam and I really need your help."

"Sure," Pam responded automatically, thinking to herself, "Why else would you be calling?" Her body sagged in the chair as she mindlessly munched on another cookie.

"I've been doing better," her younger brother went on smoothly, coolly. "I really have. Haven't touched a drop in two weeks, really I haven't. And all this isn't my fault anyway. The guy I'm staying with said I could use his couch for a while, no charge, and then after I moved in, he changed his mind. He's really pressuring me for some rent money and, if I don't pay him today, he'll kick me out."

Listening to her brother, Pam pictured the red dress she had been saving and dieting for, the one she planned to wear to her high school reunion. Her throat ached, so she took another swallow of soda. When she heard herself say, "Sure, Zach, you know I'd do anything to help you," the image of the red dress melted into the old blue one, a comfortable size larger, that was hanging in her closet. She scolded herself, "I probably couldn't lose enough weight in time to wear the red dress anyway."

"Pam, you're a doll," Zach gushed. "I knew I could count on you. What would I do without you, sweetie?"

Without answering, Pam wearily placed the receiver on the hook and stuck her hand into the cookie bag. She sat there, staring at nothing, until she had finished the entire bag.

◆ ◆ ◆ ◆

Pamela, like many sufferers of childhood neglect and deprivation, has never been taught how to attend to her own needs. To the contrary, in order to survive, she learned how to do without. Pamela concentrates on the needs of others. The oldest of four children, she was expected to care for herself and her siblings since she was old enough to change a diaper. Since both of her parents worked long hours, she has few memories of her parents at home. Pam soon learned that if she wanted dinner, she'd have to cook it herself. If she wanted to wear clean clothes, she'd have to do the wash. Adept at surviving on her own, she appeared excessively independent at a young age, for which she was constantly praised by her overworked, excessively busy parents. When her siblings arrived, one by one, it was a natural step for Pam to assume responsibility for them as well as for herself.

Recognizing Our Need For Attention

An infant, newly born with wobbly head, waving tiny hands and feet, is completely dependent on the care received from adults. If an infant is not nurtured, he or she can easily die. If you are reading this book, you can be assured that you received at least the minimal amount of touch required for survival. Many children, over the ages, have not been nearly as fortunate. Some cultures have considered exposure, leaving an infant outside to die, an acceptable form of birth control.

In the late 1800's and into the beginning of the twentieth century, American born infants had only a 50 percent chance of living past the first year of life. Children raised in institutions, of course, had an even lower chance of survival. A study of American orphans, conducted as recently as 1915, exposed the death rate of children before the age of two as high as 75 percent. The children in a Baltimore institution had only a 10 percent chance of surviving. Nearly *all* of the young children raised at Randall's Island Hospital in New York died in the institution before the age of two.[1]

Most of these infants died of a disease called "marasmus" meaning "wasting away."[2] If we look at the child-rearing practices of those times, these deaths need not surprise us. As odd as it may seem to us today, the medical community and religious leaders combined their voices in strong admonition that parents and institutional caregivers refrain from touching children. Fearing the spread of germs and moral decay, emphasis was on cleanliness and control. Nurturing, especially when expressed through touch, was fiercely opposed as a disease-spreading means of undercutting the spiritual and moral development of children.

These American child rearing practices were heavily influenced by European ideas, particularly from Germany. One of the most influential was promoted by a respected doctor and educator, Daniel Gottlieb Moritz Schreber. He summed up the antitouch bias when he wrote, "Suppress everything in the child. . . ."[3]

Claiming this deprivation was for the child's welfare, Schreber wrote:

> If the child is lifted from the bed and carried around each time he makes noises—without checking to see if there is really something wrong—and is calmed by gentleness of one kind or another, this may often lead to the appearance of the emotion of spite later in the life of the child. I

wish mothers and nursemaids would recognize the importance of this point![4]

Influenced by such teaching, Luther Emmett Holt, Sr., Professor of Pediatrics at New York Polyclinic and Columbia University, condemned any form of physical stimulation or nurturance.
Holt even went so far as instructing parents to do away with
cradles that were then plentiful in American homes for rocking
children to sleep. Instead, children were to be placed in stationary
cribs so that they would receive no physical stimulation. Babies
were to be picked up only when feeding, the times of which were
regulated by the clock, not by the child's expressed desire or need
to eat. When a child cried, parents were warned that too much
"handling" would spoil the offspring, surely resulting in moral
decay and loss of control.[5] Dr. Jules Older writes, "Good parents
and the right sort of institutions did not mollycoddle. The experts cautioned them not to handle the child too much, not to
rock her, not to pick him up when he cried, not to cuddle, comfort—not to s-p-o-i-l the little bugger."[6] The children died, un-
spoiled.

In 1928, behaviorist John Broadas Watson extended this perspective further into the twentieth century in his book, Psychological Care of Infant and Child. Watson wrote, "Never hug and
kiss them, never let them sit in your lap. If you must, kiss them
once on the forehead when they say good night. Shake hands
with them in the morning."[7] That is, of course, if the child were
still alive in the morning.

An odd thing happened that the experts didn't count on.
Children from educated homes, raised by parents who were reading the parenting books written by the experts, were dying at a
significantly higher rate than children from less educated families. The mothers who did not read these books were thankfully
ignorant of the "proper" way to raise children. Instead, these
mothers were cuddling, rocking, and holding their children. As

hard as it is to believe, it was not until the late 1940s and early 1950s that studies of marasmus were conducted to illustrate that indeed children who are not touched are much more likely to die.[8]

When we look back over history, the value of touch and nurturance may seem obvious. Lest we lull ourselves into a false sense of superiority, however, it's important to note that, while child-rearing practices may no longer be as brutal as they once were, the antitouch bias passed down by previous generations is still alive and strong. Some hospitals still whisk infants away from their mothers immediately after birth. Some still insist that the infants are fed according to prescribed schedules, set according to the adults' needs, not the babies'. In some institutions, mothers may be given a choice to feed their infants "on schedule" (regulated by the clock) or "on demand" (in response to the child's expressed interest in nursing).[9] But even this more progressive approach reveals an underlying resentment toward the infant by labeling the feeding schedule that responds to the child's need as being "on demand."

The antitouch bias remains a major force in our society, in our hospitals, in our schools, in our therapists' offices, in our support groups, and most certainly in our churches. We are a society that both craves and fears touch. Touch has been sexualized, scrutinized, and criticized. Because of our antitouch bias, most children have not received the attention and nurturance they needed. Most of us have not received the attention and nurturance we need.

Your survival depended on how you were touched and cared for when you were an infant. While much changes after your birth, many of your needs and desires stay very much the same. Ashley Montagu asserts that "evidence suggests that the human fetus is born *before* its gestation is complete."[10] He writes:

The newborn elephant and the fallow deer are able to

run with the herd shortly after they are born. By the age of six weeks, the infant seal has been taught by his mother to navigate his watery realm for himself . . . Why are human beings born in a state so immature that it takes eight to ten months before the human infant can even crawl, and another four to six months before he can walk and talk? That a good many years will elapse before the human child will cease to depend upon others for his very survival constitutes yet another evidence of the fact that humans are born more immature, and remain immature for a longer period, than any other animal.[11]

You may be out of the womb, but you are not out of the woods. At birth, you are dependent—utterly, totally, completely. Your need for food must be recognized and supplied by others. Unaccustomed to the light of day or the darkness of night, your sleep is erratic and must be aided if it is to become regular and deep. Protection from harm is solely supplied by unknown others who, for reasons of their own, choose to use their power on your behalf. From the cleanliness of your diapers to the softness of your bed, from the warmth of the arms that hold you to the nipple in your mouth, you must rely on someone else to notice you have needs and to respond to those needs.

We all come into this world as complicated, yet vulnerable, beings. While we were all born with innate abilities, how these abilities developed and were used for self-protection depended in large part on how we were touched, especially in those first days, weeks, months of life.

The amount and manner of touch our skin receives can influence our potential functioning in virtually every aspect of our adult lives. These areas include:

- our ability to think
- our potential IQ
- our vulnerability to disease

- our capacity to verbally communicate
- our ability to trust others
- our capacity to parent
- our propensity toward violent or addictive behaviors
- our capacity to enjoy sex
- our ability to relate intimately with God

In illustration, I will briefly summarize a few of the many studies conducted in these areas. For example, research illustrates that the brain, like other parts of our bodies, is still growing at birth. Consequently, early touch experiences can actually effect how *large* the brain will grow.

In a series of studies conducted on rats, researchers compared the brain size of rats who had been raised in "impoverished" environments (more isolated, less touch stimulation) with those who had been raised in "enriched" environments (in rat colonies with "toys" and other touch stimuli.) The animals were " . . . sacrificed for autopsy when the pups were between 14 and 28 days old. At 14 days, the multifamily/enriched rats had developed a somatosensory cortex [portion of the brain] that averaged 10 percent thicker than that of the unifamily animals."[12]

Dr. William Greenough, Professor of Psychology and Anatomical Sciences at the University of Illinois, has noted that isolated animals studied "consume more food than the animals in the complex environment, and they also weigh more. But their brains are smaller."[13]

Furthermore, research on rats has illustrated how touch can increase an animal's capacity to survive physical trauma. The rats in one study were divided into two groups. The first group of rats received no human touch or nurturing beyond what was necessary for feeding and cleaning of cages. This group, eventually referred to as the "irritable rats," were described as "timid, apprehensive, and high-strung . . . frightened and bewildered."

The second group was referred to as the "gentled rats" because they were customarily petted, frequently stroked and nurtured. In contrast, the gentled rats responded with "fearlessness, friendliness, and a complete lack of neuromuscular tension or irritability."

In the next phase of the study, both groups of rats were subjected to surgery wherein their thyroid and parathyroid glands were surgically removed. Within the next forty-eight hours, "79 percent of the irritable rats died, while only 13 percent of the gentled rats died—a difference of 66 percent of survivals in favor of the gentled animals."[14] While both groups of rats experienced the same physical trauma, those who had been nurtured through touch had a significantly higher survival rate.

The impact of touch on physical health is also illustrated by studies conducted on newborn animals. One study illustrated that rats handled in infancy tested higher in immunological competence than rats deprived of similar touch. Drawing from this and other similar studies, Montagu concludes that:

> Such immunological competence may be produced through the mechanism of conductor substances and hormones affecting the thymus gland, a gland which is critical in the establishment of immunological function, and also through the mediation of that part of the brain known as the hypothalamus . . . As many investigators have confirmed, handling or gentling of rats and other animals in their early days results in significantly greater increases in weight, more activity, less fearfulness, greater ability to withstand stress, and greater resistance to physiological damage.[15]

Researchers make comparisons between the experiences of animals tested and our experiences as infants. Many believe that what happens to us after birth will either support and facilitate a healthy continuation of our gestation, or our growth will be disrupted. Were you lovingly cradled at your mother's breast, nurtured, and enjoyed? Or were you left alone in a crib? Did your father hold you against his proud chest, delighted in your arrival? Or did he dangle you out in front of him unable to comfort you as you cried? Every touching experience touched you deeply, and your body still remembers.

Neglect and Deprivation

Physical neglect is a form of child abuse. It is legally defined as the "negligent treatment or maltreatment of a child by a parent or caretaker" that may result in harm to a child's health or welfare. For example, in California, two categories of neglect exist: general neglect and severe neglect.

General neglect refers to the failure of a parent or caretaker to provide appropriate clothing, shelter, food, medical care, or supervision for a child. Physical injury to the child is not necessary for a parent to be considered guilty of general neglect.

In general, a child is untouched, with body-based needs often overlooked. For example, an infant may be left crying in soiled diapers too long, leaving the skin sore and red. A toddler's cries for something to eat may be ignored, leaving the child to suffer the pangs of hunger with a sense of powerlessness. The young school-aged boy, whose father has no time to play catch with him, flounders in his physical development, growing up to feel awkward and at odds with his own body and sense of coordination. Without assistance from her mother, the pubescent girl begins menstruating, frightened and unaware of how to properly care for her personal hygiene. All too often, child neglect is body neglect, with the child being left untrained and perhaps unable to properly care for legitimate physical needs. At the root of all these manifestations of deprivation is the breakdown of the mutual relationship between parent and child.

Severe neglect refers to a parent or caretaker who does not protect a child from harm. Damage to the child may come in the form of severe malnutrition or physical exposure. A parent is guilty of negligence if the child is placed in overtly dangerous or violent situations in which, for example, a child may be sexually molested, physically assaulted or involved in drug abuse. Medically diagnosed nonorganic failure to thrive, which can lead to death, often results from severe neglect and deprivation.[16]

Children may be exposed to dangerous, overwhelming situations without proper protection or care. For example, during episodes of family violence, often both parents are engaged, leaving the children to fend for themselves. As one parent attacks the other, the child is left to cope with terror, anger, confusion, and sadness all alone. Rarely does the child have the attention and assistance needed to cope with such feelings.

Other children may be exposed to substance abuse, witnessing adults in various stages of drunkenness or the resultant inappropriate, even bizarre behavior that can occur. Then they may even be forced to deal directly with erratic behavior by becoming a prematurely responsible adult in the situation. Some parents, by selling illegal drugs, expose their children to other potentially abusive people.

Other areas of childhood abuse, such as physical abuse, sexual molestation, and emotional violation, have received significantly more attention from professional therapists and general media than has neglect. Unless an infant is abandoned in a trash can or toddlers left clinging to the center divider of a thoroughfare, we tend to view neglect as less important than other forms of childhood abuse. One reason, perhaps, is that neglect is the *absence* of what children need and therefore leaves fewer visible scars, specific memories, or tangible evidence. Neglect, however, can be just as fatal to a young child as a deadly blow to the head, just as sexually damaging as repeated sexual molestation, or just as emotionally crippling as long-term verbal assaults.

Neglect may not leave the same scars as cuts or burns. Perhaps x-rays won't show broken bones. But neglect does leave its

markings on our body maps for those skilled in accurately reading the evidence.

Strategies for Survival

To survive neglect and deprivation, many of us have developed a variety of coping strategies. These strategies served us well
as children and, in part, can account for our being alive today.
However, the methods we used to survive dangerous childhoods
can become obstacles to enjoying life as adults. Five common
survival strategies we may use to cope with neglect and deprivation are rejection of human touch, misuse of food, codependency, passive dependent behavior, and violence.

Rejecting Human Touch

It is common knowledge that infants and children who are
frightened, instinctively turn to their parents for safety, reassurance, and protection. Children recognize safety through touch—
being held, caressed, cuddled, and stroked. If the child is
embraced and protected by the parent, he or she physically re-
laxes and is calmed.

However, children develop an exaggerated need for touch if
parents withdraw from the child or physically push their children
away. This holds true for children whose parents hold them, not
with full-body, frontal contact, but off to the side in a tentative
manner. In studies conducted on infant monkeys, Dr. M. Louise
Biggar, writes, "Rather than simply withdrawing, the primate infant often tries again to approach the mother or clings to the
mother all the harder. It seems, in fact, that the immediate effect
of a mother's rejection of her primate infant is to draw the infant
toward her. The mother both repels and at some level simultaneously attracts the infant."[17] This confuses the infant, who instinc-

tively turns to and away from the same person as both the source of threat and safety.

Studies conducted on human infants confirm this finding. Initially, a rejected child will cling to the parent, intensifying a demonstrated desire for physical assurance and comfort. However, eventually the youngster, whose legitimate need for comfort is denied, will give up asking. In fact, these children will begin to push away comforting touch when it is offered to them.

In a longitudinal study conducted in Pennsylvania, parents were evaluated according to the ways they touched their infants at 12 to 18 months of age. All infants naturally reach out for their parents, desiring body-to-body contact. Researchers noted that some parents embraced their children with full-body contact. Others, however, would turn their bodies to the side, wince, or suddenly pull away from their children.

While all children initially exhibited a desire for touch, by the age of six, those children whose parents were adverse to touch no longer attempted to make any contact with other people. To the contrary, like their parents, these children now exhibited a distaste for touch and worked to avoid touch with parents or other people.[18]

How do we become "touch avoidant?" Infants who do not receive the touch they need, initially express an excessive need for touch. When they do not receive the touch desired, these infants not only give up on receiving touch, they actually learn to reject touch when available. Many children cope with the intense pain of rejection by distrusting and rejecting all human touch. If you and I did not receive the touch we needed as infants, we are prone to develop an antitouch bias. Now, as adults, we may actually push nurturing touch away when offered to us.

Research has documented that those who push away human touch, often turn instead to stuffed animals and toys. When their mothers or fathers do not assist them in self-regulating their own distress, the children may use toys and other inanimate objects for soothing. Withdrawing from human contact, touch-avoidant children tend to play in isolation, often overstimulating themselves through play activities. In a misguided effort for self-comfort, children may repetitively rock themselves, embrace hard objects, or compulsively masturbate.[19] These studies suggest that the lack of touch in early childhood may lay the foundation for compulsive, repetitive, and addictive behaviors in later life.

Adults who were neglected as children may become involved in self-neglectful and even self-destructive, over-stimulating behaviors. Unconsciously stinging from the pain of childhood rejection, we may turn away from the healing power of touch. Instead, we find more solace in activities that, at first, seem more reliable. Proud of our careers, triumphant in our sexual conquests, jubilant in our drunken fog, we may feel soothed by the pseudo-intimacy we derive from impersonal and addictive interactions. But the "hit" or "high" soon wears off.

Driven by the ever-increasing and unrelenting need for touch and attention, we need more stimulation. Instead of meeting our legitimate need for touch in truly satisfying ways, we may choose addictive relationships with food, work, sex, drugs, alcohol, or relationships. We hope our needs will be met. They are not. Our neediness increases. A panic sets in. We try harder, needing more and more stimulation to feel "touched."

Eventually, we lose sight of our original and legitimate needs for attention and touch. Completely consumed by our addictive passions, we hit bottom, unable to feel the genuine healing touch of another human being. Touch is no longer seen as nurturing, no longer viewed as a legitimate source of attention. Instead, we degrade touch by our mechanistic sexual practices, rob ourselves of nurturance through our compulsive work schedules, violate our bodies through excessive eating, numb our pain with alcohol, manipulate our feeling states with pills. Once little children, hopefully reaching out for loving touch and attention, we become cynical, frantic adults unable to feel anything at all.

Misusing Food

"Geeesh," Amy turned her head away from the mirror in disgust. "I hate my body! I am so fat!" Trying to squeeze herself into a pair of jeans, she scolded herself, "If I could only stay on this new diet, everything would be great. But I'm such a loser. I'll never look like I want to."

Food speaks the language of our bodies' most basic need—survival. Our bodies relate directly to food. When our stomachs are full or when we are hungry, we feel it in our bodies. As we prepare a meal, we can involve our bodies through smell, sight, taste, touch, and movement. We anticipate the pleasure, looking forward to the emotional nurturance and physical satisfaction. Barbara McFarland and Rodney Susong in their book, Killing Ourselves with Kindness, write "Food has become the focus of social gatherings, a passionate hobby for many people, a pleasurable experience that enhances the quality of our lives."[20]

Many adults who were neglected children feel empty inside. To fill this hollowness, some turn to food, a physical source of nurturance. Of course, this natural need for fuel and pleasure can be used illegitimately to heal childhood wounds of deprivation. Consequently, our eating patterns can become self-destructive and even life-threatening. We know that improper diet coupled with excessive or inadequate body weight can contribute heavily to a variety of illnesses, such as heart disease, cancer, stroke, and other less serious illness.[21]

Many in this country today have a dysfunctional relationship with food. An estimated 10 to 50 million Americans are overweight.[22] Some suffer from bulimia, an eating disorder primarily characterized by binge eating and then purging activities. Purging may include vomiting, laxative abuse, fasting, or rigid dieting. Overweight, average weight, or underweight, bulimics compulsively overeat, usually in secret. McFarland and Susong describe the major symptoms as:

- binge eating

- depressed moods and self-deprecating thoughts
- extreme feelings of guilt and remorse after a binge
- preoccupation with weight and food
- fear of losing control once a binge has begun
- deep sense of inadequacy, insecurity, loneliness, helplessness
- social isolation[23]

Anorexia nervosa, in contrast, is an eating disorder wherein the sufferer maintains a state of chronic starvation. Perceiving themselves as "too fat," anorexics continually lose weight to achieve a sense of peace or well-being. To these individuals, the sense of emptiness becomes so familiar that any form of nurturance may feel uncomfortable or even intolerable. When feelings of hunger arise in the body, these individuals may congratulate themselves secretly for how little was eaten on a particular day.

Whether one overeats to fill the void or undereats to perpetuate deprivation, both processes illustrate a disregard for the body's legitimate needs. As children we needed tangible responses to our bodies' tangible needs. Those whose bodies received appropriate attention to their bodies, felt loved and protected. Those whose bodies were ignored or abused, often felt unloved, rejected, and threatened. Now as adults, we may turn to, or turn away from, food as a misguided attempt to survive.

Our longing for a tangible, touchable, smellable, tasteable, feelable response to our flesh and blood needs is powerful, legitimate, and pure. However, our legitimate needs cannot be satisfied through addictive, self-stimulating behaviors, whether they be excessively self-indulgent or self-depriving.

Codependency

Luis rested his head on the steering wheel, sick with worry about his wife, Elena. She had been drinking again, he was sure of it, but there was no way to get her to admit it. He had tried to talk to her about it, and she flew into a rage, driving off with screeching breaks and dust flying.

He looked around the mall parking lot, hoping to see her car. "What if she gets into an accident or pulled over by a cop. She could get arrested for drunk driving." His head seemed too heavy to hold up any longer. "I'll never forgive myself if something happens to her."

Luis, like so many suffering from codependency, neglected his own needs in pursuit of caring for another. On the surface, a codependent may appear to be loving, compassionate, and patient. But upon examination, codependency is a self-destructive way of life.

Codependency is a term drawing a lot of fire these days. An ill-defined concept, codependency has been used so freely that anyone who acts kindly toward another risks being labeled an addict to love. Regardless of the pitfalls of the term, and the backlash against it's misuse, I believe the term is here to stay and the malady it defines is perhaps one of the most prevalent forms of self abuse active in our society today.

Melody Beattie, in her best selling Codependent No More, defines the codependent person as "one who has let another person's behavior affect him or her, and who is obsessed with controlling that person's behavior."[24] We can become obsessed with any person in our lives—friends, children, parents, clients, supervisors, colleagues—anyone we feel threatens our well being or promises us the nurturance we need.

In a longitudinal study conducted on children who were touch deprived, researchers found that a portion of the children developed "inappropriate caregiving" behaviors. Researcher Louise Biggar reports, "Children in this group seemed to become parental toward their parents, reflecting another kind of organization attachment in infancy."[25]

Codependents often ascribe to two lies: 1) If I don't do it, it won't get done and 2) Everyone else's needs take priority over mine. The first lie is rooted in a sense of excessive responsibility and grandiose power. We neglect our own needs by taking responsibility for the care of all those around us. The hope is that by giving to others, we will receive what we need in return. Unfortunately, we usually give to those who are unable or unwilling to give back to us in satisfying, nurturing ways.

The second lie, revealing a dangerously low sense of self worth, keeps us from addressing our own needs.[26] Instead, feeling responsible yet unimportant, we abuse ourselves in the way we give to others. We perpetuate the deprivation experienced in childhood by placing ourselves last in line and making everyone else's need the priority.

I believe that today's adult codependents were yesterday's neglected and deprived children. We learned to do without and to give what little we had to others in the vain hope we'd earn a little attention. As with all addictions, this strategy doesn't work. Rather, what little we had to start with is depleted, leaving us feeling all the more needy and alone.

Passively Dependent Behavior

Barry angrily stirred his coffee while Marilyn wiped tears from her eyes. "I don't know what you want from me, Barry."

"Just open up to me. Living with you is like living with a stranger," he protested.

Marilyn sighed in frustration. "I am open! I tell you everything there is to tell!"

Barry looked at her for a long time. "You really don't know what I mean, do you? You act so independent, like you don't need anyone. You certainly don't seem to need me!"

"I suppose you're right. It's too scary to need you," Marilyn acknowledged. "It's much easier to depend on myself."

Many of us have walled ourselves off from emotional vulnerability. Perhaps the greatest fear for both men and women in our society is of appearing weak and dependent.[27]

The need to deny vulnerability can be seen in many of our psychological constructs as theorists have argued, over the ages, that the human journey leads to independence and autonomy. Traditional models of development tend to describe hierarchical stages, building upon each other as specific goals are accomplished. Dependency, so traditional reasoning goes, may be considered immature, unhealthy, or even pathological.[28] We are a society that wants to believe that a "real adult" is the rugged individualist, needing no one as he rides into the sunset with his horse and his gun.

Contrary to popular belief, it is only when our legitimate dependency needs are met within the context of mutually satisfying relationships that we can become more fully functioning and "independent." As Harry Guntrip writes in Schizoid Phenomena, Object Relations and the Self, "It is hard for individuals in our culture to realize that true independence is rooted in and only grows out of primary dependence."[29]

Many of us did not have our legitimate dependency needs met when we were children. Growing older doesn't make these needs go away. Rather, we have moved into adulthood, overburdened by the demands of unmet childhood dependency needs. M. Scott Peck describes this personality as "passive dependent." In The Road Less Traveled, Peck explains:

> . . . the word "passive" is used in conjunction with the word "dependent" because these individuals concern themselves with what others can do for them to the exclusion of what they themselves can do . . . This is not to say that passive dependent people never do things for others, but their motive in doing things is to cement the attachment of the others to them so as to assure their own care.
>
> Passive dependency has its genesis in lack of love. The inner feeling of emptiness from which passive dependent

people suffer is the direct result of their parents' failure to fulfill their needs for affection, attention and care during their childhood.[30]

Driven by our legitimate but unmet childhood needs for touch and attention, we can overstress our adult relationships with unrealistic demands for affirmation and attention. Without realizing it, we may sabotage any opportunity of receiving healing love by placing excessive expectations on others. Anger, disappointment, and deprivation may be our most familiar feelings. We may lose faith that love actually has any power to heal, because we want love to "instantly, magically, concretely, and simultaneously"[31] gratify all of our infantile, though legitimate, needs. Valuing autonomy while obsessed with romance, we publicly worship icons of individualism and weep silently in secret, aching loneliness.

It is time to change our view of our journey together. No matter how old we are, no matter who much money we have, no matter how powerful we become we never outgrow our need for mutual experience. Dr. Daniel Stern, in The Interpersonal World of the Infant, asserts that all of us require the opportunity to share our emotions and experiences with others and will need to do so for the rest of our lives.[32]

Rather than view the healthy adult as the man or woman who is isolated and cut off from mutually satisfying relationships, we need to reframe our understanding and acknowledge that we will always be dependent on other people for our humanness and for the quality of our lives. The goal of our human journey into adulthood is not to learn how to be alone, separated from others. Rather, our happiness and healthy adult functioning will be marked by our ability to love each other, to share our lives and ourselves.

Mutuality is the cornerstone of our survival, of our humanity, regardless of our age. The qualities that make up enjoyable, mutually beneficial relationships hold true regardless of those involved, whether the relationship be between a gurgling infant and cooing mother, two giggling teenagers, or a romance between lovers. We all need to share our experiences, our feelings, and our lives to be healthy and alive.

I believe that on an unconscious level, we realize the power of touch for healing. And yet, if we were not touched appropriately as infants, we usually misuse touch as adults. While some become touch-avoidant as we discussed previously, others compulsively touch others in inappropriate or violating ways. Driven to feel connected to others, our neediness clouds our vision, and we literally grab for what we need.

Violence

"Is she going to be alright?" Katrina asked the nurse anxiously. "How is my baby?"

The nurse eyed Katrina suspiciously, "We are doing everything we can. How exactly did this happen?"

Katrina closed her eyes and tears squeezed out of the corner. "She, ah, fell out of her crib somehow. I don't know exactly. I was away for just a couple of minutes and, well, ah, I heard her cry. I brought her in immediately."

"As soon as I know anything more, I'll let you know," the nurse said turning toward the room where Katrina's baby girl was fighting for her life.

"Please," Katrina reached out and grabbed onto the nurse's arm. "Please save my baby. I didn't . . . I mean . . . just save her, please."

We commonly believe in this society that adults who are violent and abusive were probably abused and battered as children. And indeed, violence often breeds violence. What is less understood is that neglect also breeds violence, a physically angry response to the frustration of a need unmet.

Studies conducted on infant monkeys amply illustrate the

tremendous impact the loss of maternal touch has on these young primates. In a study conducted by Dr. Martin L. Reite, Professor of Psychiatry at the University of Colorado, monkey infants immediately responded to the loss of their mothers by searching

> ... vigorously for their mothers ... The period of behavioral agitation is accompanied by marked increases in both heart rate and body temperature, characteristic of generalized physiological arousal ... Agitation is followed in a day or two by a profoundly different reaction, distinguished by a slouched posture, little or no play behavior, a slowing of motion with evidence of impaired coordination, and a sad facial expression ... It is interesting to examine these findings in relation to symptoms of grief in human beings, since the separated monkey infants appeared to show a grief response.[33]

Similar studies demonstrate that the strongest negative impact on infant monkeys comes primarily from a loss of touch. Dr. Stephen J. Suomi, from the National Institute of Child Health and Human Development, observes that infant monkeys that are denied the ability to touch their mothers, even though they can still see, smell, and hear their mothers, no longer engage in any "exploratory activity."[34]

Monkeys that are raised in this isolated state, for at least the first six months of life, subsequently "avoid most social contact as adolescents and adults." When these monkeys do engage socially with other monkeys, they tend to be "hyperaggressive." Furthermore, as parents, these isolated monkeys tended to mistreat and neglect their own offspring. In fact, over a third of the mother monkeys in one study were overtly physically abusive to their babies. So abusive were these mothers, that the research staff had to remove the infants from the cages to insure their survival.[35]

Remember, these mothers were not victims of physical abuse,

but were victims of severe neglect and touch deprivation. This loss is so powerful, that these monkeys were unable to love their own infants. In fact, they violently responded to the needs of their infants for touch and nurturance, to the point of jeopardizing their infants' lives.

Does Your Body Remember Neglect and Deprivation?

Perhaps those painful, confusing moments of neglect are long forgotten from your conscious mind. Be assured that our bodies remember.

- Each time we push away comforting touch, our reaction speaks of past rejection.
- When we cling to others with a desperation that confuses and overwhelms us, our bodies speak of past deprivation.
- Excessive hostility, perhaps to the point of violence, may indicate a rage from past neglect.
- Hands hanging limply at our sides, no longer trying to reach out to others, may reveal hopelessness and despair.

What does your body tell you about your past experiences, neglect and deprivation? To better assess your personal body map, I urge you to spend some time answering the following questions. I also encourage you to discuss these questions with your therapist, support group, or close friends. People close to you may be able to detect clues that you might overlook.

1. Attitudes
   » What is my attitude toward touch?
   » How do I feel when someone touches me?
2. Behaviors
   » Do I receive touch from others easily?
   » Do I withdraw from others when they want to hug or touch me?

» Have I violated other people's boundaries in order to get the touch I needed and wanted?

» Do I give to others what I need myself?

» Does my obsession with others cause me to neglect my own body?

3. Body Sensations

» Do I feel all parts of my body?

» Do parts of my body feel numb or cut off from the rest of me?

» Do I feel empty inside? If so, where in my body do I feel this emptiness?

» Do I only feel my body when someone else touches me?

4. Posture

» How do I stand most of the time, in an inviting or rejecting stance?

» Do I hunch my shoulders or stand upright?

» Do I clench my jaw?

5. Breath

» What is the natural rhythm of my breath?

» In what situations do I breathe more deeply than others?

» What feelings do I experience when I change my breathing pattern?

6. Muscle Tension

» What situations cause my muscles to tense?

» Are there certain places in my body that I hold more tension than others?

» Are these areas tender or sore to the touch?

7. Body Memories

» Do I remember past experiences when others try to touch me?

» Do I avoid closeness because I fear feelings or memories I might recall?

»   Are there blanks in my memory of the past?

8. Need for Touch

»   Do I crave touch all the time, never feeling like I have enough?

»   Am I uncomfortable when other people try to touch me?

»   Do I enjoy being hugged? Would I rather no one touch me?

9. Other Evidence of Childhood Experiences

»   Do you have pictures of yourself as an infant?

»   How are you being touched in these pictures?

»   Are your parents and caregivers touching you in positive ways? Are you being touched at all?

The answers to these questions can help you discern whether or not you received an adequate amount of touch when you were a child. Your body map can also tell you if you are currently being touched in ways that are nurturing and satisfying. If your body map reveals that you would benefit from more attention and nurturance, you can chose to increase the touch you now enjoy. Through massage and body work you can receive today the touch you have always needed.

Notes

1   Jules Older, Touching is Healing, (New York: Stein and Day, 1982), 49.

2   Ashley Montagu, Touching: The Human Significance of the Skin, 3rd edition (New York: Harper & Row, 1986), 97.

3   Older, Touching, 51.

4   Morton Schatsman, Soul Murder: Persecution in the Family (New York: Random House,1973), 61.

5   Older, Touching, 98,99.

6   Ibid., 51.

7   John B. Watson, Psychological Care of Infant and Child (New York: W.W. Norton, 1928)

8 Montagu, Touching, 99.

9 Constance Maria Lillas, Quote from interview with author, 1992.

10 Montagu, Touching, 53 (my emphasis).

11 Ibid., 49.

12 Marian C. Diamond, "Cortical Change in Response to Environmental Enrichment and Impoverishment," The Many Facets of Touch, ed. Catherine Caldwell Brown, (New Jersey: Johnson & Johnson Baby Products Company, 1984), 22-23.

13 Ibid., 28.

14 Montagu, Touching, 20-21.

15 Ibid., 28.

16 Office of the Attorney General, Crime Prevention Center, Child Abuse Prevention Handbook, August 1988 rev.ed. (Sacramento: State of California, 1982).

17 Louise M. Biggar, "Maternal Aversion to Mother-Infant Conflict," The Many Facets of Touch, ed. Catherine Caldwell Brown,(New Jersey: Johnson & Johnson Baby Products Company, 1984)

18 Ibid., 67.

19 Constance Maria Lillas, "Alexithymia: Etiology and Treatment Implications for Psychoanalysis, (Ph.D. diss., Newport Psychoanalytic Institute, 1992), 42.

20 Barbara McFarland and Rodney Susong, Killing Ourselves with Kindness: Consequences of Eating Disorders. (Hazelden Foundation, 1985), 1.

21 Ibid., 6-9.

22 Ibid., 6.

23 Ibid., 2.

24 Melody Beattie, Codependent No More (San Francisco: Harper/Hazelden, 1987), 31.

25 Biggar, "Maternal Aversion to Mother-Infant Contact", 71.

26 Carmen Renee Berry, When Helping You Is Hurting Me: Escaping the Messiah Trap (San Francisco: Harper & Row, 1988).

27 Lillas, 1992, 65.

28 Lillas, 1992, 22-31.

29 Harry Guntrip, Schizoid Phenomena, Object Relations and the Self (Madison, CT: International University Press, 1969), 268.

30 M. Scott Peck, The Road Less Traveled: A New Psychology of Love,

Traditional Values, and Spiritual Growth, (New York: Simon & Schuster, 1978), 101-2.

31 Lillas, Alexithymia, 18.

32 Stern, 1985, 3-14.

33 Martin L. Reite, "Touch, Attachment, and Health—Is There a Relationship?" The Many Facets of Touch, ed. Catherine Caldwell Brown, (NJ: Johnson & Johnson Baby Products Company, 1984), 60-62.

34 Stephen Suomi, "The Role of Touch in Rhesus Monkey Social Development," in The Many Facets of Touch, ed. Catherine Caldwell Brown, (NJ: Johnson & Johnson Baby Products Company, 1984), 42,43.

35 Ibid., 44,45.

Chapter Four

Your Body Remembers Accepting Touch

"Here," Karin said, placing her four-month-old daughter in my arms, "Take care of Anna while I find my keys to open the door."

I suddenly found a squirming roll of blanket, soft flesh, and dribble in my arms. Anna and I looked at each other with shared skepticism.

Laughing at our mutual concern, Karin assured me, "You'll do fine with her. It's just a few minutes here until we get into the house."

Anna answered her mother's confidence in my ability to provide for her care with a howl that shot straight through my head, entering the ear drum closest to that little mouth and flying out the other. "Apparently," I complained as we entered the apartment, "I have yet to win her over."

"Here," Karin said, gathering her noisy child, "What's the matter, my dear one?" Anna gulped a silent swallow of air, then threw her head back and let out another pitiful cry. Smiling at me, Karin yelled over the wailing, "See? You didn't need to take this so personally. Something, other than you, is amiss here."

"That's comforting," I muttered as Karin reviewed the possible clues. Karin explained loudly, "This cry is usually her way of telling me her diapers are wet or she's hungry."

"She has different cries?" I hollered back.

"Oh, yes." Karin affirmed, unbuttoning her blouse and cradling Anna to her breast. Blissful silence filled the room. "I'm learning to pay attention to her facial expressions, her tone of voice, the way she moves." Beaming at her contented daughter, Karin said, "We know what we're saying when no one else does, don't we, Anna?"

I learned, first hand, from Anna that as small infants we have the capacity to communicate how we feel and what we want. Infants have not yet learned to separate themselves from their bodies like many adults have, but unabashedly use their bodies to let their caregivers know exactly how they feel.

Recognizing Our Need for Acceptance

Each of us is born with the capacity to experience and express nine emotions. These nine emotions are:

1. Interest/Excitement
2. Enjoyment/Joy
3. Surprise/Startle
4. Distress/Anguish
5. Fear/Terror
6. Anger/Rage
7. Shame/Humiliation
8. Contempt
9. Disgust[1]

As a newborn you were as fully able to experience body-based feelings as you are today. In some cases, infants are even more able to feel and express emotions authentically, as they haven't yet been told that certain feelings and modes of expression are unacceptable.

We do not have to learn how to feel our emotions. Rather, we emerge from the womb capable of emotional expression. Cross-cultural studies have shown that infants from all over the world are born with the ability to experience and express these nine feelings or "affect" states.

Charles Davis in his book, Body as Spirit, asserts that "feelings are bodily responses that are animated by intelligence and spiritual affectivity."[2] Babies are free to experience their internal body sensations, such as hunger, gas pain, or sleepiness, as well as exterior influences such as wetness, room temperature, or the brightness or darkness of the room. These sensations evoke one or more of the nine emotional states available to all infants. For example, hunger may trigger a feeling of distress. Warmth may result in a feeling of enjoyment. The presence of parent may stir up a sense of interest or even excitement.

Each baby reacts in his or her unique way to internal body sensations as well as exterior events. Each baby also develops a personal way of expressing these feelings. Some may cry, while others will gurgle. Rocking the head may mean enjoyment to one child, while signaling surprise in another. Each child learns to express emotion individually.

The expression of emotion is a body-based activity, both on an outward, observable level and on an internal level. Robert Timms and Patrick Connors explain this in their book, Embodying Healing:

> Most adults can easily identify the outward muscular movements sometimes used to express anger or rage. These emotions, like sadness, fear, and others, may also be expressed by inward muscular movement, contraction, a sense of retreating inward. Regardless of whether the movement is outward (pacing, screaming, crying, laughing, dancing) or inward (flushing, tightening of the throat, rising blood pressure), emotions are expressed through muscle movement.[3]

Even though we were born with the capacity to feel these nine feelings, many adults find that they are cut off from some or all of their own emotions. Researchers have found that we must "share" our feelings with others, especially during the first two years of life, in order to have access to experiencing and expressing these feelings in later years.

When we were infants, we actively tried to share our feelings and experiences with those around us. Desiring to share a new discovery or needing help in bringing a difficult feeling under control, we used our small bodies to signal those we trusted. Some of us may have communicated through our gaze, others through motion or perhaps through a gurgle, call, or cry. The goal was to find a caregiver who would share our feelings, who would become "attuned" with us.

All of us need to feel understood, and no one feels this need more strongly than an infant. A caregiver and a baby experience attunement when they *share* a particular feeling, and communicate this shared feeling in individual ways.[4]

As you might have noticed, only three of the nine emotional states are what we would consider "positive" or "enjoyable." Two-thirds of the feelings we are innately able to experience are difficult or distressing. We need our parents to attune to our feelings and help us prolong pleasurable experiences. By sharing our giggles, our gurgles, and our new explorations, our parents taught us how to enjoy positive emotions.

We also learned how to tolerate uncomfortable situations. Each time our parents soothed us as we cried or responded to our signals of distress, they taught us ways to decrease the number and duration of our unpleasant emotional experiences. As infants, we were unable to teach ourselves these vital lessons. We needed our parents to share our emotions and thereby teach us how to feel and manage our own feelings.

These are the lessons Karin teaches Anna on a daily basis. For example, Karin loves to play with her daughter. As soon as Anna stirs from her nap, Karin scoops her up with a giggle and a hug. Sharing these joyous moments together, Karin creates more than just an afternoon's entertainment. She teaches Anna how to enjoy herself and the company of a loved one.

When Anna is angry or ashamed or fearful, Karin's comforting response achieves more than a momentary, emotional salve. Anna learns how to share her pain and receive comfort, a skill she will need for the rest of her life. She also learns how to comfort herself in those moments she might find herself alone. Anna's lifelong patterns of relating to herself, her body, her emotions, and her loved ones are being set, right now, through her interactions with her mother.

As infants, we needed our parents to share our feelings and experiences with us. Those feelings that were shared, became the basis for emotional well being and expression in adult life. Dr. Daniel Stern asserts in his book, The Interpersonal World of the Infant, that affect attunement plays an important role in an infant's ability to recognize that internal feelings are shareable with others.[5]

By paying attention to their baby and the baby's body, parents learn how to accurately interpret the unique cries, coos, sighs, and movements. Each time the infant is responded to in an affirming and accurate way, the child receives so much more than mere "attention." Karin gave Anna more than a meal when she accurately interpreted and responded to Anna's cries of distress and hunger. Not only did Anna receive milk for her stomach, she also was aided in the intellectual task of linking up her interior sensation (hunger) with her feeling state (distress) and her exterior experience (breast/food/comfort). As Karin paid attention to Anna's internal sensations, emotional reactions, and exterior experiences, Anna was simultaneously learning to pay attention to herself. As her skin was touched, and the rest of her body took in this experience, this information was used by her developing brain to organize her reality. Anna's body map was being developed to include all aspects of her experience, including her mother, her feelings, her mode of expression, and, most significantly, her body.

When attuned to one another, you and your parent began to

mutually influence each other, as you first explored and then established a style of relating. Both you and your parent benefited from this mutual relationship. Judith V. Jordon in "The Meaning of Mutuality," explains that, "there is intrinsic pleasure in mutuality in relationships. This pleasure may grow from the early spontaneity and joy that exists in the mother-child/father-child interactions characterized by cuddling, hugging, babbling, smiling, 'oohs' and 'ahs.' Both participants in these early exchanges often seek to extend these engagements, and there is true pleasure and growth for both people in the back-and-forth interplay."[6]

These mutual interactions that shaped the your "self," were complex and quick. Since "the primary experience of self is relational, . . . the self is organized and developed in the context of important relationships."[7] From birth, you were able to interact with others in "split-second" timing. A particular interaction between you and your caregiver may have been brief, as you gurgled with delight, searching with your eyes of some evidence that your joy was shared. If you caught the attention of your caregiver and your happy moment was shared, both you and your caregiver benefitted from the moment. But if no eye contact was made, or you were ignored, the moment was lost.

Videotapes have been used to record mothers and their babies interacting. Microanalysis of these tapes have given us information we couldn't gather in the past. We now know that newborns and their mothers share feelings and experiences through behaviors, so tiny, that some only last a half a second.[8]

Because these interactions are so quick, most originate more from the unconscious mind than from conscious intent. Most parents impact their children less from conscious choices they make and much more from their own unconscious body maps. Through these tiny, often unnoticed interactions between us and our parents, we were shaped by unconscious forces our parents may not have recognized. Their positive intent was not enough for us to grow into healthy adults. Whatever strengths or weaknesses our parents may have recorded in their unconscious body maps were passed on to us in our infancy, in the many, minute, and often ordinary interactions we shared day after day.

Emotional Abuse

Little Andy was hungry. His tummy hurt and he wanted everyone to know it, especially his mommy. First whimpering, then breaking into a full cry, he held his head back and wailed at the sides of his crib.

"Can't you do something about that kid, Marge?" Andy's father complained to his wife.

"It's not time for his feeding," Marge responded firmly. "He's got to learn that he can't manipulate us. He'll grow up spoiled if he doesn't learn to wait his turn."

Andy rolled over onto his back, letting the tears flow into his mouth. The salty taste made him feel even hungrier. Taking a deep breath, he paused for a moment and then let out another long wail. No one responded.

Andy cried until finally his throat hurt. Exhausted from calling for his mother, his eye lids grew heavy. Whimpering, wet and sticky from his tears, he fell into a troubled sleep.

"Wake up, Andy!" His mother's voice startled him as his back arched in fear. "It's time for your feeding!" Marge reached into the crib, drawing Andy into her lap. Weary, sick to his stomach from crying, Andy weakly sucked on the bottle.

Looking over at her husband who had entered the nursery, Marge said, "See what a good boy he is? I told you it pays to show children from the beginning what's expected of them."

◆ ◆ ◆ ◆

Parents emotionally abuse their children when they disregard the wisdom of their children's bodies. Some parents are unwilling or unable to share all nine feelings with their newborn children. This intergenerational abuse is often passed on unwittingly, since emotionally abusive parents were often emotionally abused themselves as children. As a consequence of their own abusive pasts, many adults do not trust their bodies and therefore miss important messages sent their way. Parents, who are deaf to the message of their own bodies, rarely recognize or honor the wisdom of their children's bodies. Even though their children's bodies speak clearly, through inconsolable crying, irregular sleep patterns, fussiness, bouts with colic, food allergies, constipation, infections, or inattentiveness, these parents often miss the message.

Your body remembers if your parents responded or disregarded your feelings. Your body map recorded the times your parents may have considered you too young to understand, an inconvenience, or even an animal to be tamed. How you were touched deeply affected how you felt about your parents, yourself, and your body.

The term "touching" is defined in the Oxford English Dictionary as "the action, or an act, of feeling something with the hand." Touching and feeling are closely linked, both physically and emotionally. "Although touch is not itself an emotion, its sensory elements induce those neural, glandular, muscular, and mental changes which in combination we call an emotion. Hence, touch is not experienced as a simple physical modality, as sensation, but affectively, as emotion."[9]

Because the link between touch and emotion is so strong, disregarding the wisdom of the body has tragic consequences, resulting in life-changing, painful, and disruptive emotional trauma. Emotional abuse is often difficult to define, perhaps because like neglect and deprivation, there may be little physical evidence left behind. The impact of emotional abuse, however, can be as crippling as any other form of trauma, because it strikes so close to the child's sense of self and relationship with the body.

Emotional abuse impacts the body and is therefore recorded by the body. You may remember experiencing some emotionally traumatic events. Other experiences you may have consciously forgotten. While you may have no conscious memory of such damaging events happening to you, I assure you that your body remembers. Emotional abuse comes in many forms. Two of these are misattunement and ridicule of the body.

Misattunement

We are never too young to learn about feelings. In fact, from the beginning, our parents unconsciously teach us which of the nine emotions we are allowed to share. When a parent attunes to a particular emotion, we are taught that this feeling is acceptable, expressible, and sharable. However, the converse is also true. Those feelings that are rejected or ignored by our parents become isolated from interpersonal context.[10]

Some families are uncomfortable with certain feelings. For some, anger may be an unacceptable emotion. For others, fear may be unacknowledgeable. Not only are "negative" feelings considered unacceptable by some families, "positive" emotions may also be rejected. Parents may be uncomfortable when their children express curiosity or interest in exploring new adventures. Children may be taught to repress their enjoyment, instructed to be "quiet" or to face the fact that life is difficult rather than a place to play. Positive self regard may be interpreted as "conceit" or "pride," so that children are discouraged from exhibiting pleasure in their own accomplishments, interests, or talents.

Simply defined, misattunement occurs when a caregiver misses the body's message by misinterpreting, disregarding, or overriding the baby's feelings and experiences. Even the best of parents are human and therefore unable to match up with every expression, need, or feeling a child may have. Fortunately, our psyches and bodies are created to tolerate a certain amount of misattunement without being seriously impaired, but how much?

Therapists Howard Baker and Margaret Baker describe the difference between a "good enough" parent and a parent-child relationship that seriously damages the infant's emotional development. No parent can pay attention to every nuance or respond to every demand. Responsibilities of daily life, competing needs of other family members, illness, fatigue, and other obstacles may block a parent's ability to empathize at any given moment. However, for the good enough parent, these breaks in empathy are the exception, not the rule. The good enough parent is one who honors the child's body and creates a *pattern* of emotional attunement, with mismatches occurring only occasionally.

The misattuned parent, on the other hand, develops a *pattern* of mismatching and frustrating the child's efforts for closeness.[11] Misattunement results when the parent consistently misses the message. The key word here is "pattern." What makes up a positive or negative pattern of parent-child interaction?

A vital element in setting up a healthy or hurtful pattern is the parent's capacity for empathy. To empathize is to "comprehend the experience of others from their own unique perspective . . . It has both affective and cognitive elements—one feels what the other feels and then, through a complex, not necessarily conscious process, becomes aware of what the other is feeling."[12] A mother who empathizes with her child is a mother who, for the most part, pays attention and honors her child's body, feelings, and experiences.

Serious problems do not arise from an occasional "oops." Misattunement and its seriously damaging consequences occur through habitual disregard for the child's feelings, body, and well being. For example, a parent may disregard a baby's natural sleep cycle. Each of us has a personal sleep cycle, with which our fathers and mothers cooperated or fought against. Recognizing the need infants have for regulation, many parenting experts have, over the years, insisted that parents put children "on a schedule." The child suffers if this schedule is determined by outside forces, such as the parent's sleep cycle or by the arbitrary hours of a clock. An attentive parent will recognize and honor the natural rhythm of the child's body. If however, your body was not honored, your natural rhythm may be impaired.

Some parents fear that, if they follow an infant's sleep cycle, their lives will be disrupted and at the mercy of the child. Research shows that quite the opposite is true. It appears that those parents who attend to their infants' body rhythms, especially during the first week of life, get much more sleep than those who try to control their babies' sleep patterns!

Early infant researcher, Louis Sander, reported that when a mother followed her newborn's biorhythm, the infant gained a sense of directing the mother and being an active player in his or her own self-regulation. Providing the infant with a sense of importance and mastery, especially in the first week of life, had startling results. Rather than have the child's sleep cycles disrupt the household, those babies whose mothers perceived the baby as holding the timing and direction of sleep states were able to accommodate to a regular pattern of sleeping at night and being awake during the day.

However, the babies whose mothers perceived that the babies' sleep states should be regulated by the adults' control were unable to differentiate between day and night. Sleep states in these babies remained erratic. Ironically, those households where the parents tried to dominate and control their infants' sleep state were the ones most disrupted by the babies' sleep problems. Without being honored as competent human beings, these babies were unable to learn how to self regulate their sleep patterns and therefore unable to accommodate to a regular routine that assisted the family as a whole.

Perhaps what is most startling about Sander's study is that

this vital interaction takes place during the first week of life. It is critical that a newborn gain a sense of mastery between the fourth and sixth day of life. By the end of the first week, a caregiver lays the groundwork for the infant's sense of self control and establishment of sleep cycles.[13] We all have been deeply impacted by how our parents responded to us from day one.

Baker and Baker claim that "repeated empathic failures by the parents, and the child's responses to them, are at the root of almost all psychopathology."[14] The feelings that were rejected or unshared with a caretaker when we were infants may be the very emotions that are cut off from us as we grow older. Sometimes these banished emotions are "stored" in the body, waiting to be retrieved and shared.

Ridicule of the Body

The rubber band snapped, pouring Cindy's long, curly hair over her face. Cindy snarled at the mirror, "Well, at least this way no one can see your huge nose." Wiping the hair away from her face, she stared sadly at her nose. In the back of her mind, she could still hear her brothers' cruel voices screaming, "Run for your lives! The Bird Woman is here and she'll peck you to death with her beak!" Unable to tolerate their jeers, little Cindy would run away, crying, to hide in her room. There she played alone, lost in her own pretend world where she was the beautiful princess that everyone loved.

Once she overheard her Aunt Sally say to her grandmother, "Cindy would be such a pretty girl if it weren't for her nose. What a shame she had to take after her father's side of the family."

"What a shame, indeed," she repeated aloud into the mirror. "It doesn't matter how great my hair looks or what effort I may make in my wardrobe," she thought hopelessly, "all anyone ever remembers about me is the size of my nose." Letting her hair fall, tangled around her shoulders, Cindy decided, "What's the point in trying. I'm ugly and I might as well accept it." She turned from the mirror, shut off the light and walked out of the bathroom, feeling defeated and ashamed.

Like Cindy, children can be emotionally abused through ridiculing a part or parts of their body. Thinking back on my childhood, I can remember Freddy, with his thick glasses propped on his little nose, being called "Four Eyes" and Brenda, with red hair, referred to as "Carrot Head." Any body part can generate ridicule—freckles, hair color or texture, facial features, arms, legs, or behinds.

Children subjected to this form of abuse are actually "renamed" according to their source of ridicule, and may come to identify themselves, not with their full identity but as an "ugly nose," an "unacceptable foot," or an "embarrassing hairy arm." Body-related emotional abuse can come in other forms as well. For example, some children are shamed because of their gender. This form of rejection can strike both boys or girls, depending on the nature of the family dysfunction. Chris' mother prayed, once hearing she was pregnant, "Lord, if I have to have another child, then at least give me a boy." Chris was very much a girl and was rejected by her mother, because her anatomy was decidedly female.

Of course, males can be subjected to this form of abuse as well. To be unwanted due to your gender can lead to feelings of betrayal, first and foremost, by your own body, by your genitals. As soon as such a child leaves the womb and is physically inspected, the child is given verbal and nonverbal messages of being inferior, unacceptable, and unloved.

Other children, accepted for their gender, receive negative messages about themselves through their parents' reactions and feedback concerning specific developmental stages:

◆ ◆ ◆ ◆

"Steve just isn't as coordinated as his older brother, Jack.

Why, when Jack was Steve's age, he was running all over this house. Poor little Steve is just getting the hang of crawling. Who knows what will become of him?"

"Diana! I can't believe you wet the bed again! What do I need to do with you? Hang the sheets outside so everyone can see what a bad little girl you are?"

"Skip, put that down! Stop getting into everything! Can't you just sit still for a minute? I work hard all day and come home to a wild monster like you. You're going to be the death of me!"

◆ ◆ ◆ ◆

Children who are not allowed to develop physically and emotionally at their own pace are often shamed and punished for behavior that is normal and appropriate. Unfortunately, these children receive distorted messages about who they are and about the acceptability of their bodies.

Some victims of emotional abuse do not experience such overt verbal attack or emotional rejections of their bodies or bodily functions. Yet, children who are shamed, through ridicule of their bodies or through other means, carry the impact of such trauma within their bodies:

- the little girl who endures the verbal abuse of an alcoholic father may slump her shoulders forward as a physical expression of "guarding her heart."
- the ten-year-old boy who feels responsible to care for his siblings, may develop tension in his shoulders as his body responds to "carrying the world on his back."
- the teenage girl, who fears rejection of her mother, may try to hide her growing breasts so as not to threaten her mother's sense of womanhood.

Even though a survivor of emotional abuse may never experience the bodily pain of being hit, raped, or deprived of needed nurturance, the body becomes the reservoir of pain, remembering the shame, recording the ridicule, and expressing the feelings the child is unable to say.

Strategies for Survival

In order to deal with emotional abuse, we develop a variety of strategies for survival. Strategies include living in fantasy, desperately seeking attention, hating our bodies, or seeking the perfect body. Consider the following:

Living in Fantasy

Cindy, ridiculed by her brothers for the size of her nose, was overwhelmed by shame. In addition, she felt unprotected and ridiculed by the adults in her life. Consequently, Cindy concluded she had no one who could help her.

Because she did not know how to deal with difficult situations effectively, Cindy turned away from the outside world, choosing instead to create a fantasy world, one that numbed the pain and promised to give her the nurturance she needed and desired. Sitting for hours by herself, she would pretend she was a beautiful princess who was held captive by a cruel dragon. All the knights in the kingdom risked their lives for her and the chance to gaze at her beauty.

Other children use a variety of fantasy escapes. These may include excessive television viewing, incessant reading of comic books or other fantasy material, or overly investing in a particular hobby. These activities can be positive in themselves but can be an indication of serious emotional pain if excessively utilized.

Desperately Seeking Attention

While some, like Cindy, seek to escape their pain in the world of fantasy, others become excessively invested in pleasing others. Desperate for the affirmation they need, emotionally wounded children may go to great lengths to get attention. Often talented, outgoing, and sensitive, such a child may become involved in drama, musical performances, or athletic accomplishments. It is not uncommon to see these children overly stress their bodies to out-perform other children their age.

Desperate for attention, it is vital to stand out in a crowd. Being "average" will not gain the attention needed. Insecure in their own skins, they do not live in a relaxed, creative manner. Rather, these children feel driven to earn their worth.

Seeking the Perfect Body

"Look at these abs!" Cindy beamed, lifting up her t-shirt to show Sandy, her workout partner. "I've worked on these all summer and they are finally getting into decent shape."

"Great . . . job. . . . Cindy . . . " Sandy puffed between reps. "I told you that you could make your body look just the way you wanted, didn't I?"

Cindy eyed her rump. A frown came over her face. "Yes, you did. But I'd be so much happier if my body believed you as much as I did. I was so humiliated last weekend at the beach. My thighs are atrocious."

Sandy sat up from the weight machine. "Then stop talking and start working out, girl. Take control of that body. Don't let it control you!"

Many children who have suffered emotional abuse hate their bodies or the parts of their bodies through which they experience criticism. As a young girl, Cindy learned to hate her nose, and held this part of her body responsible for the ridicule she suffered. Like Cindy, these children turn on themselves, blaming, not the emotionally abusive individual, but the body part that is criticized. At an early age, children can come to hate their faces, their hands, their feet, their hair, their eyes, or even their entire bodies.

As Cindy grew older she began to hate, not merely her nose, but the rest of her body as well. In fact, few American adults are pleased with their bodies. Surveys have revealed some alarming results:

- Over 50% of Americans claim to be unhappy with their weight or the size of their abdomen.
- Thirty-eight percent of women and 34% of men are unhappy with their physical appearance.
- In 1990, a whopping $33 billion was spent on diets in this country.
- Muscle-building equipment brings in $750 million annually.[15]

Motivated less out of healthy self care and more out of a hatred of the body, this society is obsessed with compulsive dieting and excessive exercise. Those who are emotionally alienated from their bodies often relate to their bodies as machines, to be sculpted and molded at will. Robert Chianese warns:

> Fitness seekers, if they rely exclusively on remaking their physical selves for both self-defense and self-fulfillment, ultimately shrink their emotional selves. They sever their connections to others, and place an impossible burden on their bodies to be the sole source of rest and renewal. In a valiant but misguided effort at self-empowerment, they may wind up cut off from, and helpless before, an ever more threatening world. The fitness seeker may become a victim of self-inflicted, panicky isolation.[16]

So dissatisfied are some with their bodies, that over a million and a half Americans are electing to undergo cosmetic surgery each year. As we enter the last decade of this century, we find 75,000 Americans getting their faces lifted, over 100,000 are altering their noses, and more than 130,000 women are getting breast implants.[17]

Some are even resorting to genetic engineering techniques to assure their children will have a better body. Across the country, some parents are electing to have their children injected with a human growth hormone because they are *short*! Aware that this treatment is potentially hazardous to their children's health, these parents are responding to the pressures of a society that worships the tall and thin. Andrew Kimbrell writes, "With the advance of genetic engineering, we may be gaining the ultimate weapon against the body, a final solution that ensures victory over our stubborn flesh, blood, and bone."[18]

Body-hatred shows itself in subtle, yet powerful ways. For example, my body becomes an "it" rather than a part of me. My possession, rather than my companion. A servant rather than a teacher. Chainese asserts, "Without full acceptance of the body, there's no genuine love of self and others . . . Working the body out as a high-tech possession commits a form of murder on our human integrity, estranging the worried self from its physical form. Having torn the self from the body, we wind up denying both our body and our self the right to a healthier social and natural environment."[19]

Emotional abuse can follow us into adulthood if we believe our bodies are to blame for our pain. Long after those childhood years' experiences, we can continue to emotionally abuse ourselves. Like Cindy, we become our own abuser, separating ourselves further from the wisdom of the body.

Does Your Body Speak of Emotional Abuse?

We may have consciously forgotten those tactile experiences that shaped our inner beings, our ability to comprehend the world, and our understanding of ourselves, but our bodies remember.

- Each time we flinch when someone reaches out to lovingly hug us, our bodies are signaling us that something has frightened us in the past.
- Each time our skin "crawls," our bodies are warning of us an undesirable experience, past or present.
- Each time we engage in self-abusive behavior, such as overeating, alcohol abuse, addictive sex, compulsive work, codependency, or lack of self-care, we betray our lack of respect for our bodies.
- Our slouching posture speaks of sadness, hopelessness, unresolved pain, or excessive weariness.
- The tightness in our hands, lower back, and neck speaks of the week's tension and stress.
- The knots in our calves, back and shoulders carry the memories of emotional abuse endured years ago.

In order to help you better decode your body map, I invite you to become more aware of the ways your body speaks to you in these ways:

1. Attitudes
   » What is my attitude about my body?
   » Do I trust my body?
   » How can I better respect my body?
   » How did childhood experiences shape my attitudes about my body?
2. Behaviors
   » Do I engage in self-destructive behaviors?
   » Do I overeat? overwork? misuse drugs or alcohol? engage in self-abusive sex?
   » Do I get the rest I need?
   » Do I exercise and eat properly?
3. Body Sensations

» How does my body communicate with me about stress? illness? sadness? joy?

» Does my stomach churn when I'm anxious?

» Do I get headaches when I'm under too much stress?

» Do any parts of my body feel numb?

» Does my eye twitch when I'm angry?

» How can I better express the feelings my body carries?

4. Posture

» Do I sit or stand in a self-protective stance? aggressive manner? fearful posture?

» Do I clench my jaw?

5. Breath

» Do I tend to hold my breath, or do I breathe deeply and calmly?

» Do I have a shallow breath pattern?

» Do I tend to gasp for breath?

6. Muscle Tension

» Where do I carry tension in my muscles?

» What feelings do I feel when I relax?

» How do these knots in my muscles feel when pressed? numb? painful? sore? pleasurable?

7. Body Memories

» Do certain types of touches, smells, sights, sounds or tastes trigger memories from the past?

» Are there blanks in my memory of the past?

» Do memories tend to frighten or comfort me?

» Are parts of my body more sensitive to touch than others? Are some parts numb? others extra sore?

8. Need for Touch

» Do I feel satisfied with the amount of touch I am currently receiving? Do I tend to shy away from people who want to touch me? Do I feel that, no matter how much I am touched, it's never enough?

◆ ◆ ◆ ◆

Has emotional abuse separated you from your body? Only you can answer these questions with any certainty.

If you realize that, indeed, you view your body with suspicion and distrust, I urge you to make peace with your body. Your body, no matter what anyone has ever told you, is trustworthy and wise. As you learn the special symbols of your body map, you will better understand what has happened to you in the past and how best to address needed emotional healing. A major component of healing from emotional abuse is reconciling yourself with your body.

Notes

1 Tomkins' study is described by Virginia E. Demos, "Affect and the Development of the Self: A New Frontier" in Frontiers in Self Psychology, ed. A. Goldberg. Vol. 3 (NJ: The Analytic Press, 1988), 29.

2 Charles Davis, Body as Spirit: The Nature of Religious Feeling (New York: The Seabury Press, 1976), 9.

3 Robert Timms and Patrick Connors, Embodying Healing: Integrating Bodywork and Psychotherapy in Recovery from Childhood Sexual Abuse (Orwell, VT: The Safer Society Press, 1992), 26.

4 Daniel Stern, The Interpersonal World of the Infant (New York: Basic Books, 1985), 6.

5 Ibid., 156-57.

6 Judith V. Jordon, "The Meaning of Mutuality," in Women's Growth In Connection: Writings from the Stone Center, (New York: The Guilford Press, 1991), 87.

7 Janet L. Surrey, "The Self-in-Relation: A Theory of Women's Development" in Women's Growth In Connection: Writings from the Stone Center, (New York: The Guilford Press, 1991), 52.

8 Daniel Stern, "A micro-analysis of mother-infant interaction: Behaviors regulating social contact between a mother and her three-and-a-half-month-old twins," Journal of American Academy of Child Psychiatry, 10, 1971, 501-17.

Daniel Stern, "The first relationship: Infant and mother," Cambridge, Mass.: Harvard University Press , 1977.

B. Beebe and D. Stern, "Engagement-disengagement and early object experiences," in Communicative Structures and Psychic Structures, eds. M. Freedman and S. Grand (New York: Plenum Press, 1977)

9   Ashley Montagu, Touching: The Human Significance of Skin, Third Edition (New York: Harper & Row, 1986), 128.

10 Daniel Stern, Interpersonal World, 6,8.

11 Howard S. Baker and Margaret N. Baker, "Heinz Kohut's Self Psychology: An Overview," American Journal of Psychiatry 144:1 (January 1987), 3.

12 Ibid., 2.

13 Louis Sander, "The Event-Structure of Regulation in the Neonate-Caregiver System as a Biological Background for Early Organization of Psychic Structure," in Frontiers in Self Psychology, Progress in Self Psychology, Vol. 3, ed. Arnold Goldberg, (NJ: The Analytic Press, 1988), 64-77.

14 Baker and Baker, Heinz Kohut's "Self Psychology," 2.

15 Andrew Kimbrell, "Body Wars: Can the Human Body Survive the Age of Technology?" Utne Reader, May/June, 1992, 53,54.

16 Robert Chainese, "The Body Politic: Can Fitness Buffs Become a Force for Social Change?", Utne Reader, May/June 1992, 69.

17 Kimbrell, "Body Wars," 53.

18 Ibid., 56.

19 Chainese, "Body Politic," 71.

Chapter Five

Your Body Remembers Safe Touch

Cameron's shoulders were throbbing, but he hardly noticed as he drove through the rain. With his large hands clenching the wheel, he growled to the empty seat beside him, "I can't believe I let my dad get to me again! Man!" he slammed his fist against the dash board with a bang.

The sound startled him. The watery road seemed to disappear as the image of a little body, huddled, underneath the living room end table snapped into his mind.

"Boy?" His father's angry voice filled the room like a rushing tidal wave. "You are such a momma's boy. Come out here, and take your punishment like a man. NOW!"

The only movement Cameron could produce was to tremble in terror. He knew that if he showed himself, his father would beat him. But hiding from his dad would only make it worse. There was no way out, no place to hide.

"Ah, there you are!" A large hand grabbed Cameron's little ankle and dragged him out onto the living room rug. "I'll teach you to run away from me, you little sissy!" Cameron hid his eyes as his dad took off his belt. Cameron tightened up every muscle in his body and held his breath to brace himself against the pain that was coming. Clenching his jaw, Cameron swore to himself, "I'm not going to cry. I won't even feel it. I'll never let him know how much it hurts."

The flashing of headlights from an oncoming car jarred Cameron back into the present. "Just once," he thought to himself, rubbing his shoulder with one hand and steering with the other, "I'd like to deck that guy. But I refuse to let him know how I feel."

The anger subsided as a piercing pain shot down his neck to that familiar sore spot between his shoulder blades. "Whatever could be wrong with my back?" he asked himself. The anger melted into a wave a fatigue. "Guess I'm just getting old."

Recognizing Our Need For Safety

Like Cameron, our bodies remember times when we were touched in ways that hurt or frightened us. In our muscles, we carry the fear, rage, and helplessness experienced when overpowered by those who meant us harm. From conception, we struggle to survive the various challenges and threats to our safety. Our desire to live is inborn and powerfully drives us throughout our existence.

Even within the womb, we are already aware that our survival is not assured, instinctively moving our bodies in the direction of safety. As our various sensory organs develops, we use these senses prior to birth to protect ourselves. For example, by using ultrasound, researchers watched seven-month-old fetuses respond to different sensory experiences. First, a buzzer was sounded about 18 inches from the mother's abdomen. The fetuses' entire bodies jumped, startled by the noise. All sucking motion ceased. The buzzer was sounded several more times. As the fetuses learned that there was no major threat, the startled physical response diminished. By the fourth buzzer, the fetuses displayed no response and by the fifth buzzer, sucking resumed.

Not only are we able to detect sound while in the womb, we also use our sense of sight to determine nurturing or dangerous stimuli. To test this, researchers flashed different kinds of light on the mother's abdomen. As with the previous experiment, the fetuses initially jumped, taking their hands from their mouths and looking in the direction of the light. But by the fourth flashing light, the fetuses closed their eyes or looked away, returning their thumbs back to their mouths.[1]

These experiments tell us several things about ourselves. First, we do not wait until birth to utilize our bodies' senses for self-protection. As soon as a sensory capacity develops, we use our newly gained ability to protect and nurture ourselves.

Second, these experiments reveal how we use the sense of touch to help comfort and orient ourselves. Some researchers believe that in the womb we comfort ourselves by sucking our thumbs. This hand-to-mouth activity helps us orient ourselves to new and possibly threatening experiences.[2]

Early childhood experts T. Berry Brazelton and Tiffany Field write, "Touch provides the baby with an adaptive and containing opportunity by helping him handle sensory and motor overload ... Autonomic and central nervous system development begin before birth; touch and containment are at the base of the learning that accompanies their development."[3]

"Touch" and "containment" are key concepts to understanding our need for safety. Through touch we come to define our "containers." Often referred to as "boundaries," these containers define "what is me and what is not me. A boundary shows me where I end and someone else begins, leading me to a sense of ownership."[4] Through our early experiences with touch, we learn whether or not our containers safely define and protect us from harm.

Our most basic self-defining boundary is our skin. Therapists Henry Cloud and John Townsend write, "The skin boundary keeps the good in and the bad out. It protects your blood and bones, holding them on the inside and all together. It also keeps germs outside, protecting you from infection. At the same time skin has openings that let the 'good' in, like food, and the 'bad' out, like waste products."[5]

Our sense of safety is often influenced by the manner in which our physical boundaries are honored. As an infant, your body helped you protect yourself in several ways.

First, your skin lets you know a great deal about the person touching you. Were their hands warm and inviting or cold and anxious? Was your skin stroked with affection or ignored? Were you treated gently or harshly? It is through the use of factors such as "pressure, intensity, rhythm, duration, firmness, and the like, that infants are able to discriminate between those who, when holding them, care for them and those who do not."[6]

How our skin is touched communicates clearly about our safety and well being. As an infant, you were able to detect whether or not the person touching you intended you good or ill. As amazing as that may seem, as a newborn you were not only able to detect the physical sensation of touch but also the intent of a person's touch.

Our bodies are able to detect levels of care, unconscious motivations, and conscious intent. In response to dangerous situations, our bodies respond automatically through changes in body temperature, heart rate, breath rhythm, muscle tension, and voice quality.

Second, you were acutely aware of who picked you up, how kindly or harshly you were held, and how the person felt about you when they touched you.[7] Your muscle-joint-ligament movement, or "proprioceptors," signalled you about the safety of a situation, letting you know how safe you were by the way others held you. Were you held securely or loosely? Gently or too tightly? Was the person who held you relaxed or anxious, annoyed or pleased? Were you welcomed or unwanted? This information impacted your emotional development. Was this new world safe or scary? Were you loved or a bother? Could you count on these people or not?

Montagu asserts that infants, held by adults who are tense, anxious, or threatening, can develop hypertensive habits. "These hypertensive habits later show up in hypertensive conditions affecting the gastrointestinal tract in the form of colitis, hypermobility, ulcers, and the like, affecting the cardiovascular system in the form of psychogenic cardiovascular disturbances, affecting the respiratory system in the form of asthmatoid conditions, and, of course, affecting the skin in a large variety of disorders."[8]

Third, our ability to anticipate how the people in our lives will respond to us aids in our survival. Some might believe that the ability to anticipate another person's behavior or an event is too sophisticated for an newborn. Not so.

Even though our bodies are still growing in size, complexity, and capacity, we come into this world as competent individuals. Infants are able to detect predictable experiences. In fact, we require predictability in order to develop physical and emotional well being. Our caregivers' predictability and the predictability of positive experiences and events were central to our overall intellectual and psychological development. So important is this pattern of "predictable sequences"[9] that some researchers claim that all other dimensions of our development are dependent upon this critical interaction.[10]

To illustrate this, I'll describe a series of experiments. One of the things babies do best is suck. The experiments were designed to see if babies could be taught to use their sucking rhythm to "turn on" music by changing their sucking motion. In the first experiment, babies learned that, if they paused between sucking bursts, music would start to play. Researchers noticed that, when the music played in line with expectations, the babies appeared pleased.

In the second experiment, the babies initially were taught to turn on the music through changing their sucking rhythms. The babies in the second experiment also appeared pleased. But then, their expectations were violated. The researchers did not turn on the music to correspond with the babies' behavior; instead they played music randomly. This frustrated the babies. Some grimaced and whimpered. Others cried. Some of the babies stopped sucking all together.

In a final experiment, a new group of infants were exposed to the randomly played music. Then researchers tried to teach the babies to start the music through modifying their sucking rhythm. Startling as it may seem, the babies in the third group were unable to learn this task. Once they experienced a violation of anticipation, their capacity to learn was seriously impaired.

Being able to predict what will happen to us impacts our ability to learn and our capacity to feel safe in the world. From conception, we are concerned with interacting with others in predictable and safe ways. If those around us share our concern and work with us to protect and honor our expectations, we are free to grow up emotionally relaxed and spiritually open. Our bodies function to their optimal levels, providing us with health and a sense of well being. However, if our expectations are violated, all areas of our functioning suffers.

Physical Abuse and Trauma

Birth Trauma

All warm and snugly, you were delighted by the soothing and stimulating caress of your mother's womb. You floated with plenty of space and no competition. Then one day, without warning, you were squeezed down a narrow passage that pressed against your head and upset your plans for the afternoon.

Grabbed by unfamiliar hands, you were whisked away from your dark, quiet cocoon into a noisy swirl of bright lights and probing fingers. Screaming in surprise, you sucked in your first breath of air, startled at the sound of your own voice. While everyone else in the room may have considered this your "birth," you may have very well wondered if this new and strange experience might not be the death of you.

The birth experience, at best, is physically taxing, and our familiar world radically alters. Prior to birth, we expect life in the womb to continue. We have nothing to warn or prepare us for the catastrophic change of moving from an "aquatic solitary existence into an atmospheric and social environment."[11] Montagu explains:

> At birth, atmospheric air immediately rushes into the lungs of the newborn, inflating them and causing them to press against and to produce gradual rotation of the heart. There is, as it were, a competition for space between the heart and the lungs. The ductus arteriosus between the arch of the aorta and the upper surface of the pulmonary trunk, which in the fetus made it possible to bypass the systemic circulation involving the lungs, begins to contract and close. The cupulae of the diaphragm begin to rise eccentrically up and down, the chest wall to expand, all of which could hardly be described as contributing to a pleasant experience for the newborn.[12]

Without warning, we lose our soft, warm, and safe container and find ourselves alone and unprotected. Until recently, most babies were separated from their mothers immediately following birth, placing the hospital's procedural needs over the needs of the children or mothers to be together. Birthing practices are now taking the needs of the mother and child into consideration, creating a less traumatic, more nurturing transition.

While vaginal birth is inherently traumatic, this experience provides infants with the most positive manner to arrive into this life. The pressure, caressing, and pushing the infant's body receives during vaginal birth contributes to overall functioning. Cesarean-delivered babies often experience a number of disadvantages over those who are born vaginally. The mortality rate is higher among cesarean-delivered babies, some estimate two to three times as great. Death from hyaline membrane disorder, a respiratory complication, is ten times more frequent. In a comparison study conducted by Dr. Gilbert W. Meier of the National Institute of Health, vaginally delivered babies were "more active, more responsive to the situation, and more responsive to additional stimulation" than were cesarean-delivered babies.[13] No matter how we come into the world, we have tremendous obstacles to face . . . and our bodies remember the trauma of birth.

Physical Abuse

Physical abuse is first and foremost an assault on the child's *body*. Through the infliction of physical pain and bodily damage, the child experiences the abuse. Fists bruise the child's delicate skin, blackening eyes and bloodying the nose. Swinging belts rip into the soft tissue of arms and legs and buttocks. Bones snap. Cuts bleed. Burns blister. These physical offenses are inflicted on the child's body, with seriously damaging consequences.

When a parent or caregiver physically assaults a child, the adult uses the child's body as a weapon against the child. The parent hurts the child by hurting the child's body. The child's body and psyche experience pain through hitting, burning, twisting, kicking, or pushing. The adult abuser can bruise the child's spirit, break the child's sense of safety, and twist the child's self esteem into self hatred.

Western society has taken quite a while to recognize the negative impact physical assault has on a child. For centuries, parents have been admonished to use harsh physical punishment to discipline children. In fact, for the greater part of human history, children were considered "property" rather than persons.

For example, in ancient Babylonia, infants were not granted the right to live by virtue of birth alone. Survival required acknowledgment of the father. An unacknowledged child was immediately killed.

Roman and Greek cultures echoed this disregard for a child's right to live for centuries. A major shift occurred in the fourth century, when church leaders, "in line with the Judaic commandment, 'Thou shalt not kill,' equated infanticide with murder. This was a landmark in the history of children's rights."[14]

The attitudes we have in the United States regarding children and the treatment given to their bodies have been most strongly influenced by English laws, specifically the English Poor Law established by the Crown in 1604. For the first time, the government assumed responsibility for the poor in its jurisdiction, including the children. Prior to this time, parental rights were the only rights acknowledged and honored. Here we see that children, and their bodies, are recognized as having rights of their own.

The belief that parents "own" their children and answer to no one for their actions, however, is deeply ingrained in this society. In fact, Americans established the Society for the Prevention of Cruelty to Animals *before* efforts were made to protect children from parental abuse.

A historic shift in our understanding of proper child treatment occurred in 1871 when a young girl named Mary Ellen was heard screaming night after night from her New York home. Concerned church workers contacted local authorities to stop the beatings of this poor child. At that time, however, society had no mandate to intervene between a parent and child. Finally, the church workers called upon the Society for the Prevention of Cruelty to Animals, arguing that Mary Ellen was a member of the animal kingdom and deserved as much protection as a dog or cat. Finally, the SPCA intervened and a new phase of child protection effort came into being.[15]

Another historic shift occurred nearly a century later when Henry Kempe, a pediatrician at Colorado Medical Center, drew international attention to what he called, the battered child syndrome.[16] Physicians began to study suspicious cuts, bruises, fractures, and other physical damage suffered by children that had previously been attributed to accidental causes. In the past few decades, we have come to see that physical abuse perpetrated by caregivers is prevalent, listed as one of the major causes of child death in our country.

Physical abuse leaves its mark on every aspect of the child's being. Certainly, physical scars can remain after the burns, breaks, and cuts have healed. The body remembers these offenses at a deeper level as well, through shallow breathing, hunched shoulders, fearful glances, clenched teeth. In studies conducted at the National Center for Post-Traumatic Stress Disorder, researchers found that "even one experience of overwhelming terror permanently alters the chemistry of the brain. The longer the duration and the more severe the trauma, the more likely it is that a victim will develop PTSD."[17]

PTSD, or post-traumatic stress disorder or syndrome, is a common response to physical abuse. The symptoms include, but are not limited to, "amnesia, nightmares, and flashbacks. People who have PTSD may 'leave their bodies' during the abuse, and they may continue to dissociate for decades after the abuse ends."[18]

Strategies for Survival

Since physical abuse is a direct assault on our bodies and therefore a direct threat to our survival, finding strategies to deal with this type of abuse can be a life or death matter. Children may respond to the pain of physical abuse by becoming numb, holding in the pain, or perpetuating the violence.

Becoming Numb

We all survive by avoiding pain and pursuing pleasure. Children, with minimal options, try to protect themselves from harm as best they can. When children realize they are unable to protect themselves from pain by getting way from an abusive situation, some children try to protect themselves from pain by "getting away" from their bodies. For some, this means literally numbing themselves to bodily pain or pleasure, cutting themselves off from feeling most physical sensations.

As a body worker, I have worked with many clients who claim to feel nothing whatsoever in their bodies. Heather is such a person. The survivor of an alcoholic mother with violent mood swings, Heather initially felt nothing as I worked on the many large knots along her neck and shoulders. "Go deeper! No one who's worked on me ever goes deep enough," she would complain. "I want to feel something."

I could sense that I was pressing into her muscle tissue at a deep level, with further pressure possibly resulting in bruising. It was not, as Heather initially believed, the lack of pressure that kept her from feeling her body. In order to protect herself from the physical pain of her childhood abuse, she had separated herself from the sensations of her body.

This skill aided her in surviving her childhood, and as a child, it served her well. As an adult however, this survival skill impeded her ability to respond to actual pain in her body and, worse yet, to enjoy the pleasure she could receive through her body. As we worked together, and her trust in the safety of our relationship grew, so did her ability to feel body sensations. Within a few months, we shared a chuckle over her complaining, "Ow! You're going too deep! Those knots in my shoulders are sore!"

Holding in the Pain

Some of us cope with child physical abuse by holding the pain inside our bodies. Cameron learned to protect himself from his father's angry outbursts by hiding his feelings and taking his beatings "like a man." As a little boy, Cameron became adept at holding his breath and his feelings. Right before a beating, he would tighten his arms and shoulders, burying his feelings deep within the muscle tissue. Now, as an adult, when he begins to feel rage, he unknowingly assumes a cowering body position as the muscles between his shoulder blades contract. Cameron has yet to accurately read his body map when his muscles throb with years of unreleased tension. Instead of feeling his anger directly, Cameron sinks further into a sense of helplessness and fatigue.

I am in no way advocating that Cameron, or any survivor of abuse, use violence as a means of healing. It is critical, however, that our bodies be allowed to release the tension, the pain, the memories that we have stored within them day after day, year after year. Body work and massage present effective and safe means for this release. Touch was the vehicle for abuse for many as children. Now touch, as adults, can be the vehicle for healing.

When we allow our bodies to release stored tension through body work and massage, we also open ourselves up to the feelings we were unable to deal with as children—fear, anger, helplessness, sadness, betrayal, confusion. Now as adults, we can learn new survival skills that include, rather than exclude, our bodies.

Perpetuating the Violence

Violence perpetuated by children and teenagers has become an everyday experience, seen nightly on the news. Reports of children hurting other children and animals confronts us regularly. Children are being taken into custody after attacking or even killing their parents, claiming their violent acts are self-defense due to suffering abuse at their parents' hands.

Years ago, I worked as a house parent in a residential center for abused children. Most of the children in our care were survivors of serious physical abuse. I remember Melody, an eight-year-old girl, thin and wiry, who had been repeatedly beaten by her mother until she was removed from her home at the age of six. While I was on duty one afternoon, Melody flew into the living room, enraged by an argument she had with her school teacher.

Rather than control her angry impulses, Melody picked up a large, heavy, metal chair. I was utterly amazed that this tiny girl had the strength to lift that heavy weight. I was even more surprised when, flooded with adrenaline and rage, Melody then threw this chair across the room and over the couch. Her anger gave her additional strength, and the potential ability to do a great deal of harm.

Melody is one of many young children who learn to use violence as a way to express their feelings. Pumping their bodies with adrenaline, their muscles contract their hands into fists to hit and harm others. Legs learn to kick, teeth are used as weapons as the body is turned into a means of violence rather than nurture and love. Abuse begets abuse. Unfortunately, a child is never too young to learn a lesson in violence.

Does Your Body Remember Childhood Physical Abuse?

We may consciously remember times in the past in which we were physically violated. It is also possible that we were abused but these memories are no longer available to the conscious mind. Instead, our bodies may remember.

- Each time we duck when a friend warmly extends a hand to pat us on the shoulder, our bodies remind us that not all hands are safe.
- The way we hold our breath and watch intensely in fear when a particular type of person comes into view may indicate that someone with similar characteristics hurt us in the past.
- Having difficulty feeling body sensations may be our bodies' way of revealing our attempt to avoid physical pain.
- Our tapping toes and clenching fists may indicate unidentified anger stored in the body.

- Assuming an overly confident or "macho" posture may speak of hidden fear due to past abuse.
- Outbursts of violent behavior including breaking objects, hitting walls, or assaulting others may reveal our own violated vulnerability.

The following questions may help you get a more accurate reading of your body map.

1. Attitudes
   » What is my attitude about my body?
   » Is anger a common experience for me?
   » Do I rarely feel angry for fear I might explode and hurt someone else?

2. Behaviors
   » Do I treat my body with respect?
   » Do I treat other people's bodies with respect?
   » Have I used my body as weapon to hurt others?
   » Have I assaulted anyone?

3. Body Sensations
   » Do parts of my body feel numb?
   » Are there painful knots and points of tension in my body?
   » Do I often clench my fists or lock my jaw when I feel angry?
   » Where in my body do I feel fear?
   » Where in my body do I feel anger?

4. Posture
   » Do I sit or stand in a fearful posture?
   » Does my body look as if it is ready to fight? to run? to duck?
   » How do I hold my arms?

5. Breath
   » Do I tend to hold my breath, or do I breathe calmly?
   » How do I breathe when I feel in danger? How often do I use that particular breath pattern?

» How do I breathe when I feel angry? or sad? or un-protected?

6. Muscle Tension
» Where do I carry tension?
» When I relax, what feelings come over me?
» Am I able to relax my muscles, or am I in a constant state of alert?
» Do I feel sensations in my muscles when they are pressed? What are these feelings?

7. Body Memories
» Do certain colors, tastes, smells, or sensations trigger memories of physical abuse?
» Are there blanks in my memory?
» Do my childhood memories tend to comfort or frighten me?

8. Need for Touch
» Do I push touch away or feel comfortable when I am close to others?

If someone near me raises their hand, do I automatically flinch assuming they are about to hit me? Do I assume they are reaching for something and mean me no harm?

Do I feel satisfied by the touch I receive?

Am I afraid to be touched, or do I feel safe when close to someone else?

Has physical abuse placed a barrier between you and your body? That barrier can be broken down and a positive relationship with your body can be reestablished. The choice is yours. Hostile, hurtful touch may have caused the damage, but healing, helpful touch can repair the past.

Notes

1 Nine Guzenhouser, Advances in Touch: New Implications in Human

Development (NJ: Johnson & Johnson Baby Products Company. 1990), xiii.

2 Ibid.

3 Ibid.

4 Henry Cloud and John Townsend, Boundaries: When to Say YES and When to Say NO, (Grand Rapids, MI: Zondervan Publishing House, 1992), 29.

5 Ibid, 33.

6 Ashley Montagu, Touching: The Human Significance of Skin, Third Edition (New York: Harper & Row, 1986), 107.

7 Ibid., 107-8.

8 Ibid., 109.

9 Beatrice Beebe and Frank M. Lachmann, "Mother-Infant Mutual Influence and Precursors of Psychic Structure," in Frontiers in Self Psychology, Progress in Self Psychology, vol. 3, ed. Arnold Greenberg, (NJ: The Analytic Press, 1988), 5.

10 L.W. Sander, "The Regulation of Exchange in the Infant-caretaker system and some aspects of the context-content relationship in Interaction, Conversation, and the Development of Language, eds. M. Lewis & L. Rosenblum, (New York: Wiley, 1977).

11 Montagu, Touching,

12 Ibid., 70.

13 Ibid., 62-3.

14 Samuel Radbill, "A History of Child Abuse and Infanticide," in The Battered Child, 2nd edition, eds. Ray Helfer and Henry Kempe, (Chicago: The University of Chicago Press, 1980), 14.

15 Jules Older, Touching is Healing (New York: Stein and Day, 1982), 66-7.

16 Ibid., 67.

17 Heidi Vanderbilt, "Incest: A Chilling Report," Lear's Magazine, February 1992, 6.

18 Ibid., 6.

Chapter Six

Your Body Remembers Intimate Touch

Wendy sneaked up behind her husband and slipped her hands around Craig's waist. Instead of relaxing into her arms as she expected, she felt his back arch as he gasped and held his breath.

In that instant, Craig recalled a scene he had long forgotten, of himself as a little boy, maybe six or seven. Craig is standing by the doorway when Gretta, family friend and frequent afternoon baby- sitter, comes up behind him and wraps her arms around his tiny waist. At first Craig giggles as she tickles him gently. But as he pulls away, she holds him tightly. A sense of dread spreads down the back of his neck as he feels her breath, warm against his tender skin.

Her hands tug at his shirt, easily finding their way inside. He arches his back in fear as she reaches into his pants. He gasps, holding his breath, too frightened and confused to speak. His body starts to tingle as she fondles him. His toes curl downward as he clenches the carpeting.

"Doesn't that feel good?" Gretta whispers. Craig, too frightened to breathe, can't answer. Abruptly, she pulls her hands from his pants and swings him around to face her. "You must never tell anyone about this," her usually smiling face is now fierce. "Promise me!" Gretta demands.

Craig stares at her, motionless, his back still arched, his toes frozen into tight curls.

"Promise me!" Gretta shakes him, snapping his head back.

Craig gulps for air. "I promise," he whispers. "I'll never tell anyone."

"Craig?" Wendy stared at her husband, bewildered. "Craig, what's happening with you?"

"What?" Craig responded, vaguely aware of his wife's presence as he returns from the memory of his past.

"Craig, dear," Wendy said softly, "I'm sorry if I startled you. I didn't mean to upset you. Tell me what's bothering you."

Taking a deep breath, Craig smiled sadly, "I'm not sure I can talk about it." Craig looked down and noticed his toes were curled, tightly holding onto the carpeting for fear that, if he let go, he'd float into the sky and burst into a thousand pieces like a lost balloon.

Recognizing Our Need for Intimacy

Sexual intimacy is, at its core, body intimacy. Skin touches skin, lips and tongues meet, fingers caress, and muscles tingle with electric ecstacy. Our longing for physical intimacy begins before birth and, through each phase of life, takes on different forms and expressions. Ashley Montagu writes, "The basic language of sex is tactile, not verbal. Words and images can be poor imitations of the deep complicated feelings within us."[1]

Full sexual intimacy is based on more than our physical apparatus. Satisfying sexual intimacy engages our entire selves— our bodies, minds, souls, spirits, emotions—and invites the full participation of our partner. We must learn the language of sexuality. As James Nelson writes in his book Embodiment, "The process by which we become sexual seems to be less a natural unfolding of biological tendencies than a social learning process through which we come to affirm certain sexual meanings in our interaction with significant others."[2]

If, as infants, we were insufficiently tutored to speak the language of touch, as adults our capacity to communicate through sexual, largely nonverbal means can be seriously limited. Montagu emphasizes the importance of touch on our sexual functioning when he writes:

> It has been remarkable that in the final analysis every tragedy is a failure of communication. And what the child receiving inadequate cutaneous stimulation suffers from is a failure of integrative development as a human being, a failure in the communication of the experience of love. By being stroked, and caressed, and carried, and cuddled, comforted, and cood[sic] to, by being loved, the child learns to stroke and caress and cuddle, comfort and coo, and to love others. In this sense love is sexual in the healthiest sense of that word. It implies involvement, concern, responsibility, tenderness, and awareness of the needs, sensibilities, and vulnerabilities of the others. All this is communicated to the infant in the early months of his life.[3]

Our capacity to be sexually intimate as adults can be traced back to our early infant experiences with our parents, building on the shared moments of intimacy only our bodies now remember.

Sexual Abuse

Our sexuality suffers when our bodies suffer. One cannot be separated from the other. Too often we make the mistake of jumping over the physical aspects of sexual abuse, focusing instead on the emotional or even "sexual" trauma involved. It is critical that we recognize that the most basic element of sexual abuse is the violation of the *body* as boundaries are touched, probed and penetrated in ways that are beyond our emotional and physical capabilities.

Some sexual molest is seductive and soft, with caresses and kisses stimulating feelings of pleasure. Other forms of sexual abuse are crude and cruel, resulting in physical trauma to the child's body as adult-sized genitals or other objects are inserted into tiny vaginas and anuses. Regardless of the level of violence used in any sexually abusive incident, the child experiences serious trauma due to the loss of control and choice over his or her own body.

This form of body abuse is all too prevalent in American society. Nearly twenty years ago, when this society denied the existence of childhood sexual abuse, Dianna E. H. Russell, professor at Mills College, conducted a study that revealed 38 percent of the participating women had been sexually abused prior to the age of 18.[4] After a decade and a half of professional experience in child sexual abuse treatment and prevention, I now believe that sexual abuse may occur to a third, if not a half, of the children in the United States. Boys are as vulnerable to abuse as girls. As more adults come forward, acknowledging their childhood experiences, the stereotype of "female victim and male offender" no longer holds as the norm.

Mike Lew, therapist and author of Victims No Longer, claims as many as 50 percent of child victims may be boys.[5] One study estimates that 46,000 – 96,000 boys are molested each year in the United States, although a mere 7,600 cases are reported in a typical year.[6]

Boys and girls, of all ages, are being sexually violated by both men and women, who may be trusted family members, church leaders, caregivers, or strangers. Sexual abuse has a powerful impact on the child's body, regardless of gender. The body suffers in many ways.

First, the body may be damaged through physical violence perpetrated on the child during the sexual act. Sexually violent assaults result in scarred tissue, damage to sexual organs and other related physiological functions. Children have suffered injuries to the urethra, penis, vagina, anus, and mouth. In severe cases, bones have been broken, tiny bodies have been crushed, and even deaths have occurred.

New horrors confront us as we recognize the potential destructiveness of sexually transmitted disease. Some have become sterile due to the physical damage of the sex act or because of the long-term effects of sexually transmitted diseases. Mike Lew writes, "Sadly, we are going to have to pay increasing attention to the issue of incest generated AIDS. Not all children who are HIV-positive were infected by birth."[7]

Second, the body suffers from sexual abuse through the violation of body-based boundaries. When the body's boundaries are violated, so are many other boundaries that are indelibly linked to the body. Emotional, spiritual, sexual, and intellectual boundaries are all affected. Therapists Henry Cloud and John Townsend claim that sexual abuse survivors "often have a poor sense of boundaries. Early in life they were taught that their property did not really begin at their skin. Others could invade their property and do whatever they wanted. As a result, they have difficulty in establishing boundaries later in life."[7]

Rather than learn how to discern and protect their boundaries, sexually abused children often survive by teaching themselves how to endure abuse. Roland Summit, M.D., professor of psychiatry at Harbor-UCLA Medical Center in Torrance, California, explains that, "the one thing a child learns from sexual abuse is how to be abused."[9] Heidi Vanderbilt concurs, "instead of learning to protect themselves, they learn they *can't* protect themselves."[10]

Third, children suffer from sexual abuse through gender and sexual confusion. Both girls and boys are negatively impacted by sexual abuse. The impact of abuse can be determined by a number of factors, one of which is the gender of the molester. Girls molested by men often respond differently than girls molested by women. Girls molested by males tend to generalize this abuse to all men. Some become sexualized prematurely, using their sexuality as a "bargaining chip" in relationships. Some withdraw from sex altogether, others deny their sexuality by hiding their bodies through dress or by putting on excessive weight.

Girls molested by women are confronted with a confusing dilemma as they find the danger, not in men as is generally expected in this society, but in a "mother figure" (if not their actual mother). Since girls establish their sexuality by identifying with their mothers and other adult females, abuse by a woman can seriously disrupt this natural process. Janet L. Surrey in "The Self-In-Relation," explains, "A good relationship is highly valued by both mother and daughter and becomes a fundamental component of women's sense of self-worth . . . Within the early mother-daughter relationship, the daughter is encouraged to learn to take the role of the mother (or, we could say, the 'provider,' the 'listener,' or 'surround' [sic]) as well as the daughter (the 'receiver,' the 'speaker,' or the 'figure') . . . This mutual 'care taking' is a fundamental aspect of learning."[11]

If the boundaries of this vital relationship are violated through sexual abuse, the daughter learns not how to care for another but how to hurt and abuse. The girl molested by a women is confronted with two self-violating choices: to deny her own body and sexuality by rejecting femaleness or to embrace her body and find herself somehow a member of an abusive class of women.

Boys also suffer from childhood sexual violation. While we as a society assume that girls can be victimized, we are reluctant to see males, even small boys, as vulnerable. We assume that characteristics of masculinity include "macho, robust, muscular, athletic, strong, vigorous, lusty, powerful, potent, and fearless."[12] Characteristics like "vulnerable," "frightened," and "small" just don't come to mind. Thanks, in part, to the men's movement, male sexual abuse survivors are feeling more able to acknowledge they were molested as children.

Therapist Mike Lew writes, "Men are simply not supposed to be victimized. A 'real man' is expected to be able to protect himself in any situation. He is also supposed to be able to solve any problem and recover from any setback. When he experiences victimization, our culture expects him to be able to 'deal with it like a man.' Unfortunately, 'dealing with it like a man' usually translates as avenging the hurt (preferably violently) and then forgetting about it—moving on."[13]

For a small boy, who is not yet a man and yet feels the same expectations, sexual victimization can be an isolating and overwhelming experience. Unsettled in the meaning of their sexuality, these boys struggle alone with their confusion and fear. Asking for help would, of course, be unmanly.

If the molester is a female, the boy faces other forms of confusion and isolation. A male victim experiences all the pain, confusion, grief, horror, and loss as would any child who is sexually victimized. However, in this society, we have a distorted view about sexual activity between a boy and an adult woman. Insisting that males are the aggressors and females the prey, regardless of the age, our society romanticizes this form of sexual abuse. The boy is supposed to enjoy his "conquest" rather than grieve his loss of innocence.

In his work with male survivors of child sexual abuse, Mike Lew reports:

> It is my impression that male survivors are more likely to repress memories of abuse by women than by men. It is not uncommon that previously forgotten or particularly occluded incest memories are recovered in the safety of an incest recovery group. Memories of female perpetrators seem to be more resistant to recovery[;] when they do come up, they appear to be more devastating and more emotionally damaging.[14]

Male and female survivors have some common struggles.

The body retains the physical recording of the smells, tastes, sights, touches, and sounds of the sexual trauma. These records, often referred to as "body memories," are held in body, even when the incident may be blocked from conscious awareness. Body memories are stored safely within the body, until the time may come when the conscious mind is ready to remember.

A sense of shame, especially in regard to the body, is a characteristic of both boys and girls who have been sexually violated. But we needn't be a sexual abuse victim to suffer from body-based shame related to sexuality. In addition to overt childhood sexual abuse, many children are wounded through the dysfunctional ways their families, friends, and society at large respond to sexuality and sexual expression. Just as children can be shamed about their bodies through childhood emotional abuse, children also can become estranged from their own sexuality and appropriate bodily functions through verbal and nonverbal messages of shame and disrespect.

Growing breasts, the appearance of pubic hair, the size of one's penis, the changing of the voice, or the onset of menstruation can be the focus of ridicule. The natural need for affection and intimacy, expressed through sexual avenues, can be covered with the stench of shame and falsely placed guilt. There are few among us who cannot recount at least one incident where, as children or adolescents, we felt criticized, humiliated, or even rejected due to our body's burgeoning sexuality or sexual interest.

Strategies for Survival

What does a small child do to survive the overwhelming trauma of childhood sexual abuse? How does the little boy make sense of the feelings of helplessness? How does the little girl cope with feeling dirty and used? Where do these little ones go to grieve their losses? their pain? their confusion? How have so many in this society survived this all too prevalent childhood experience?

Common responses to sexual violation include the confusion of pain and pleasure, dissociation and repression, and use of the body as "currency" to get what one needs. Let's look more closely at these responses:

Confusing Pain and Pleasure

When we are born, we naturally pull away from pain and embrace pleasurable sensations. Sex, when experienced within age- appropriate and relational boundaries, is intended to be pleasurable. Unfortunately, when children's bodies are violated sexually, what was meant to be pleasurable, is mixed with terror, confusion, and pain.

Defending against the pain of violent assault, survivors of physical abuse may lose contact with positive physical feelings. Survivors of sexual abuse are doubly affected, in that they may cut themselves off from their bodies to avoid both the pain and the pleasure experienced during the abuse. Perhaps one of the most painful sources of guilt for the survivor of childhood sexual abuse is the acknowledgment that the abuse may have "felt good." Craig cried as he told his therapist, "I am such a bad person. I remember getting erections and even having orgasms when Gretta would fondle me." His shoulders sagged, "I'm so ashamed to admit I enjoyed any of this terror."

Children, like Craig, have difficulty sorting through the pleasures and pain, comfort and terror, caring and deception. Because sexual abuse is body abuse, many of these children come to confuse pain and pleasure, unable to distinguish harmful sexual experiences from pleasurable, positive ones. Incapable of discerning dangerous situations from safe, some may become powerless to protect themselves from further harm. In fact, some children may grow up attaching pleasure to painful experiences, unconsciously perpetuating their violation into adulthood.

Dissociation and Repression

Sexual abuse treatment expert, Dr. Elaine Westerlund, writes, "Children who are sexually abused are known to rely primarily on two defense mechanisms to cope with the trauma: dissociation and repression . . . Dissociation allows the child to manage the event(s) of victimization by separating intolerable feeling, physical sensation, and/or experience of self from the event(s). Repression is another way to cope with trauma by allowing the child to 'forget' that the abuse ever occurred."[15]

In a recent study of 43 adult survivors of incest, Westerlund reported the following findings:

> . . . dissociative responses were reported by the partici-
> pants as the most common defense during the incestu-
> ous abuse. In this study, 77% of the participants reported
> psychically "numbing" themselves, 70% reported physi-
> cally "numbing" themselves, 51% reported leaving their
> bodies, 40% reported observing themselves from nearby
> at the time of the sexual abuse event(s). As adults, 53% of
> the participants continued to rely on dissociative states
> as a means of coping . . . 85% of the participants re-
> ported having repressed all memory of incestuous abuse.
> Most women were in the late twenties or early thirties
> before memories began to surface, and most experienced
> a lengthy period of active memory retrieval (many, many
> months to several years).[16]

As these findings illustrate, many children survive molest by hypnotizing themselves during the experience, often pretending to be someone or somewhere else. The conscious mind dissociates from the actual experience, storing the memory in the unconscious mind and within the body. Often references to the "inner child" are describing that part of the psyche and the corresponding body memory which have been separated off to protect the child from the debilitating consequences of abuse, often sexual abuse.

Even children who remember their abusive experiences clearly may harbor, within their bodies, a more comprehensive impact of the abuse. Sexual abuse survivors may hold their bodies rigidly, breathing quick shallow breaths. Others may walk on the sides of their feet, unable to fully connect to the ground or a full sense of reality. Some may numb parts of their bodies, especially those parts that may be considered "sexual" in order to cut themselves off from the memory of abuse.

Carolyn J. Braddock, a noted therapist who integrates breath, sound, and movement work with talking therapy, identifies three main body types of women who have been sexually abused: rigid, inanimate, or collapsed. The rigid types have difficulty with movement and a sense of bodily freedom, as if they were tied up in knots. The inanimate body is lifeless, emanating a sense of hopelessness. Parts of the body may be cut off from feeling sensations. The collapsed body seems to be trying to become smaller, in an effort to hide from another blow, often like an animal cowering before a master.

These bodies certainly reflect a past history, a roomful of memories. It is important to include the body in the recovery process when the comprehensive impact of the abuse is this great.[17]

Using the Body as Currency

Children whose bodies are used to inappropriately gratify the sexual and power needs of adults are taught that the body is an object to be used. Some children accept this message and learn to use their bodies as a means to survive. Children of any age or gender can learn to exchange sexual pleasure for whatever they might need—affection, attention or affirmation. Some children agree to sexual involvement for material goods such as toys, food, or money.

Little Craig, fearful of retaliation from his baby-sitter, learned to trade his body and his silence for a fragile sense of safety. Often victims of incest report that they endured sexual abuse perpetrated by either or both of their parents in an effort to keep the family together. Since the child's body is treated with disrespect, an object to be used, the child may survive by cooperating with or even initiating abusive situations in order to get what he or she may need.

As difficult as it may be to conceive, some children survive their own abusive experiences by abusing other, more helpless children. Racked with rage, fear, and confusion, these children, some as young as two or three years of age, reenact their abuse by sexually seducing, molesting, and even raping other children. Both boys and girls are capable of sexually abusing other children. Unable to digest their own feelings of helplessness or anger, these little ones attempt to rid themselves of their pain by passing it on to others.[18]

Does Your Body Remember Childhood Sexual Abuse?

Memories of child molest may be clear in our minds. Or, our conscious minds may have pushed away these memories, leaving our bodies to hold the secrets.

- When certain fragrances or odors trigger a sense of panic or outrage, our bodies are signalling us of past associations.
- By recoiling from an intimate encounter or finding our bodies have no feeling when touched, we may illustrate past abuse.
- An inability to protect ourselves from sexual exploitation

as adults directs us to look at past lessons in
victimization.

- Gender confusion or conflicting sexual feelings points to childhood experiences void of clarity and acceptance.
- Feeling ashamed of our bodies, especially of our genitals, indicates past experiences of humiliation and rejection.

Certain smells, such as the cologne or body odor of the offender, may trigger a body memory. A touch, similar to the abuse, or a sound or color, may signal the body to bring into consciousness the once-forgotten horror. To more fully understand what your body map has to convey about your childhood sexual development, I invite you to consider the following questions:

1. Attitudes
   » What is my attitude about sex?
   » How do I feel about my genitals?
   » How have my childhood experiences shaped my attitudes about my sexuality?
   » Do I feel obligated to perform sexually in order for people to like me?
2. Behaviors
   » Do I engage in self-destructive sexual behaviors?
   » Do I cut myself off from sexual enjoyment?
   » Am I free to express myself sexually in a satisfying way?
3. Body Sensations
   » How does my body feel sexual arousal?
   » Am I relaxed with my sexual feelings, or do I feel anxious or distressed about sexual sensations?
   » Do I get headaches, stomachaches, or other aches when I become sexually aroused?
   » Do parts of my body feel numb?
   » Do I feel separate from my body when I become sexually aroused?
4. Posture

» Do I carry myself upright, or do I try to hide my sexual attractiveness?

» Do I sit or stand in a relaxed or a self-protective stance?

» Do I exhibit characteristics of a rigid body type? inanimate body type? collapsed body type?

5. Breath

» Do I breathe comfortably?

» Do I breathe with short, shallow breaths?

» Do I hold my breath?

6. Muscle Tension

» Where do I carry tension in my body?

» What feelings surface when I relax?

» Am I especially tense in my lower back or chest areas?

7. Body Memories

» Do certain sensations trigger memories of past sexual abuse?

» Can I remember my childhood, or are there blanks in my memory?

8. Need for Touch

» Do certain types of people frighten me, causing me to pull away from them physically?

» Do I feel that men are more dangerous than women? Women than men?

» Are there certain types of people with whom I feel more comfortable touching? What kinds of touch do I long for most?

» Has sexual abuse separated you from your body? If you were molested as a child, your body can be your guide to breaking free from a painful past. Exploitive touch may have damaged your sense of sexual safety, but now you can utilize healing and nurturing touch to achieve the restoration you deserve.

Notes

1 Ashley Montagu, Touching: The Human Significance of Skin, Third Edition (New York: Harper & Row, 1986), 204.

2 James B. Nelson, Embodiment: An Approach to Sexuality and Christian Theology, (Minneapolis: Augsburg, 1978), 29.

3 Montagu, Touching, 216.

4 Heidi Vanderbilt, "Incest: A Chilling Report," Lear's Magazine, February, 1992, 52.

5 Ibid., 53.

6 John Sebold, "Indicators of Child Sexual Abuse in Males," Social Casework: 68(2), (February 1987), 75-80.

7 Mike Lew, Victims No Longer: Men Recovering from Incest and Other Sexual Child Abuse (New York: Harper & Row, 1986), xiv.

8 Henry Cloud and John Townsend, Boundaries: When to say YES and When to Say NO, (Grand Rapids, MI: Zondervan, 1992), 34.

9 Vanderbilt, "Incest," 56.

10 Ibid., 56.

11 Janet L. Surrey, "The Self-in-Relation: A Theory of Women's Development," in Women's Growth In Connection, ed. Judith V. Jordon, et. al. (New York: The Guilford Press, 1991), 57-58.

12 Mike Lew, Victims, 36.

13 Ibid., 41.

14 Ibid., 59.

15 Elaine Westerlund, "Memory Retrieval, Management, and Validation in Incest Survivors" (Cambridge, MA: Impact Resources, Inc., 1988), 1.

16 Ibid., 1.

17 Carolyn J. Braddock, Body Voices: Using the Power of Breath, Sound, and Movement to Heal and Create New Boundaries. (Berkeley, CA: PageMill Press, 1994).

18 Toni Johnson and Carmen Renee Berry, "Children Who Molest: A Treatment Model," Journal of Interpersonal Violence, (June 1989).

Chapter Seven

Your Body Remembers
Integrating Touch

"Don't tell me," Carl's angry voice cut through Terri like a knife, "you've got another one of your headaches. At least you could come up with something original!"

Terri's fingers massaged her pounding temples as tears of frustration and pain came to her eyes. "Oh Carl. Please . . . "

"Don't patronize me," he snarled, snatching his pillow from the bed. "I can't stand sleeping next to you another night."

Terri watched her husband disappear into the hall. Throwing herself onto the bed she cried into her pillow, "Why do I get these headaches whenever he starts to make love to me? This isn't the way I thought marriage would be." Her head throbbed and her heart ached. "What is wrong with me?"

Recognizing Our Need For Wholeness

As infants, we naturally accepted ourselves, exploring our bodies with delight. We were thrilled by the discovery of our fingers, our toes, our genitals, unaware that some body parts were considered more "acceptable" than others. As adults, however, we may believe that parts of ourselves are fine. Too few of us, unfortunately, feel loved in our entirety.

We all long to be loved and accepted completely. Since we are spiritual beings, for us to feel acceptable, we often sense that this means being acceptable to God. And, since we are physical beings, this acceptance must include our bodies, our entire bodies.

I believe that our ability to express ourselves as loving, whole beings is based on our perception of others' acceptance of us. In previous chapters, we have discussed the importance of feeling touched and nurtured by others, perhaps most importantly by our parents. But even our parents cannot provide us with love and acceptance that reaches our deepest needs. I am known in the deepest places, the hidden recesses of my soul only by God. Only God can attune to us so fully as to overcome our shame and convince us we are completely loved. As theologian Paul Tillich declared:

> It strikes us when our disgust for our own being, our indifference, our weakness, our hostility, and our lack of direction and composure have become intolerable to us. It strikes us when, year after year, the longed-for perfection of life does not appear, when the old compulsions reign within us as they have for decades, when despair destroys all joy and courage. Sometimes at that moment a wave of light breaks into our darkness, and it is as though a voice were saying: 'You are accepted. *You are accepted* . . . Simply accept the fact that you are accepted!' If that happens to us, we experience grace.[1]

How do we experience this grace? How do we see this wave of light? How do we hear this accepting voice?

Divine acceptance and love is communicated to us through a variety of avenues: inspiration through nature, insight through dreams, intimacy through prayer, guidance through sacred writings, solace and serenity through meditation, encouragement through relationships. Through these means and others, we can sense the presence and intimations of a divine presence in a way that makes us feel like we have been touched.

One of the most significant avenues of spiritual communication is through our own bodies. While many spiritual traditions pit the body and spirit against each other, I believe that honoring the body is an integral part of our spiritual path. Since our bodies are created by God, our bodies reflect God's nature and character. From observing our bodies, and enjoying our physical selves, we learn many things about spiritual life.

Our innate desire to survive illustrates that God is a lover of life. Our bodies come equipped with instinctive, self-protective impulses. Through conscious responses and automatic reflexes, our bodies sustain and protect us. And when we are hurt, our bodies are equipped with self-healing capabilities.

While God is believed to be everywhere at all times, our bodies reveal to us that we are also separate from God and that our privacy is respected. Our bodies, specifically our skin, delineate where we begin and end. As philosopher Maurice Merleau-Ponty writes, "My understanding of my body is the key to my understanding of bodies and places beyond me."[2] Through our physical boundaries, we find our definition, our identity, and our reference point in the world.

Our body boundaries do not isolate us from others. Rather our boundaries make it possible for us to be intimate with other separate personalities. We long to know we are not alone. Our own cravings for touch and closeness, certainly a positive valence in creation, reveal that spiritual intimacy is possible. Through the ages, mystics, rabbis, monks, and ordinary people from all religious traditions have shared a longing for intimacy with the divine. I believe this desire, experienced within the body, tells us about God's own desire for closeness with us.

Our sexual organs and erotic desire tell us about a divine creative love. Creative potency and intense passion bespeak a Creator who is fully conversant with our existence, with bodies full of sexual desire. Only a God who revels in pleasure could create the many nerve endings, soft skin, the erogenous zones, and the genitalia required for full-body sexual enjoyment.

If we include our bodies in our spiritual journey, we can learn these and many more spiritual truths. But if we degrade the body, rather than view it as a divine creation, we overlook important information about divine love. We must use our eyes to see, not only our face in the mirror but also a reflection of the divine face.

Our bodies not only reflect a spiritual character. The everyday workings of our bodies become spiritual receptors through which God communicates to us. As living, breathing, desiring, growing, changing, loving, physical beings, our bodies are designed to receive spiritual communication on a regular basis. For example, we are warned of too much stress through our back pain and headaches. We are guided to people who are safe through our relaxed body posture or informed of danger through our sweaty palms or shortness of breath. We are called to rest through droopy eye lids and energized to play through a pounding, excited pulse. Our desire for intimacy is affirmed as our bodies respond to passion and sexual desire. Our entire bodyselves are a delight and celebration of the Divine Presence who loves us.

I believe God values us greatly and is offended by our mistreatment. As a consequence, our bodies are designed to register misattunement or trauma. Our physiological makeup could have easily been constructed to forget the past, whether positive or negative. Instead, I believe our bodies are designed to record all that happens to us so that future healing is possible. Nothing about us is unimportant. Nothing about us is lost. Our bodies remember.

Our lives are significant. Your life is significant, as is your body and everything about you. Love is communicated to you, through the delicate blood cells that course through your veins, through the muscle tension in your shoulders, through your sexual longings, through the beating of your heart, through each breath you take into your lungs. It's as clear as the nose on your face—you are loved and offered grace every minute of the day.

Spiritual Abuse

Unfortunately, grace may not be a common experience in all of our lives. Rather than feeling wholly loved, our lives may be splintered by past assaults on our bodies, our feelings, and our spirits. While all forms of abuse are hostile to the body, spiritual abuse is perhaps the most damaging to our sense of wholeness, because it severs our bodies from our spirituality.

As I have studied the many faces of abuse, I have been stunned to find that religious writers from all traditions are some of the most outspoken and unyielding opponents of the body. In spiritually abusive religious circles, this attitude is common, and rarely subtle, as spirit is unabashedly separated from and elevated above body. This tragic violation of our wholeness is usually touted as a spiritual virtue.

Until I included my body into my spiritual journey, I believed my thoughts were superior and more trustworthy than my feelings. Spirituality was "up" and the body was "down." I'd been taught to enhance my spiritual walk by decreasing my concern with "earthly" things which meant anything to do with my body.

I am not the only person detrimentally affected by distorted spiritual teaching. Many of my body work clients suffer damage due to a body-mind split. Since spiritually abusive ideologies avidly elevate the spirit over the body, such religious teaching has historically warned against any association with the body. Reflecting our interior division, we come to see the world in terms of dichotomy. As James Nelson writes, "We become resistant to ambiguity and seek simple, single reasons for things. Our conceptual worlds become populated with dichotomies—me/not me, male/female, masculine/feminine, heterosexual/ homosexual, black/white, smart/stupid, healthy/ill, good/bad, right/wrong." [3]

Consequently, spiritually wounded people are almost always at odds with their bodies. Rather than experience our bodies as illustrations of a creative and loving grace, our physical selves often trigger bouts of shame. Theologian Alexander LaBrecque observes, "A lot of us have been taught theologically that to think badly of ourselves is a spiritual thing to do." Specifically critiquing certain Christian traditions, LaBrecque states, "In some quarters of the Christian church, a test of orthodoxy is how badly one thinks of humanity." [4]

A spiritually abusive faith demands that we illustrate our spiritual superiority by exhibiting our low self regard. For example, one client, a seminary student named Peter, was referred to me for help by his therapist because of his irregular eating patterns. Peter, close to fifteen pounds below the recommended weight for his height, refused to eat whenever he felt badly about himself, which, unfortunately, was much of the time.

As Peter allowed me to touch him in nurturing ways and to respect his body as a source of spiritual guidance, he realized that his distorted religious beliefs were a threat to both his spiritual and physical health. He told me, "Instead of eating I would pray for hours and hours, begging God to tell me what to do with my life. Now I can see that by ignoring my body, I was pushing away God's guidance."

As Peter heals from the spiritual abuse he's suffered, the animosity between his body and spirit decreases. He still devotes time to prayer, but now he also eats regular, nutritious meals. Peter smiled when he said to me, "I can pray *and* eat! It's not an either-or situation. In fact, now I love God not only with my spirit, but with my whole self—my body, mind, and soul!"

Peter discovered an important spiritual truth: Healthy spirituality unifies rather than divides. Abusive spirituality drives us further from a divine connection, not closer. Normal physical functions cause us to hide ourselves in shame rather than bond us closer to God in intimate passion. In our efforts to hide our bodyselves, we forget how to be fully present. Instead of living as whole persons, spiritually wounded people are partial people, splintered by shame.

Severing the body from the spirit also severs our minds from the grounding nature of the body. We ignore the still small voice when it comes by way of our bodies. Without the needed "reality checks" provided by the body, the mind is free to float and create distorted dogmas. A particular idea may be "logically consistent," and thereby accepted as truth by the mind, but prove to be false in a flesh-and-blood world. Intoxicated by exaggerated self-importance, the disembodied mind reasons, unencumbered by the body's reality. As a consequence, toxic paradigms have contaminated our spiritual heritage, further barring us from receiving divine communication through the body.

While "splitting" a person into two competing parts may have been touted as a religious virtue over the years, psychological studies illustrate that the process of splitting is an extreme, self-mutilating response to an intolerably painful or threatening experience. " . . . In situations of acute bodily terror, the psychic sense of 'being' can be protected by seeming to be separated from the physical body. This preserves the sense of 'being' and guards against the dread of 'not- being.' . . . In very insecure children . . . the psyche and the soma have seemed to be split apart. Before they were equipped to do so, they have had to take responsibility for their own sense of 'being.' "[5] Without divine love we become "insecure children" indeed. Spiritually, many of us have become like the child hiding in the corner with her eyes closed, pretending no one can see her.

The important guidance God gives to us every day through our bodies goes unnoticed. I remember times when I accused God of forgetting me as I overlooked the many ways God was communicating to me through my body. By distrusting my body I lost contact with a viable and reliable source of spiritual guidance.

Strategies for Survival

Spiritual abuse leaves us warring against ourselves. In order to survive this unnecessary war, we may cut ourselves off from our sexuality, cut ourselves off from God, or become a body worshipper.

Cutting Ourselves Off from Our Sexuality

While other forms of abuse degrade different aspects of our physical selves, spiritual abuse tends to express its particular brand of body hatred by stigmatizing sexuality. The Christian church, in particular, has erred by dividing body from spirit and then overly eroticizing the body.

Perhaps this confusion is due, in part, to the close link between spirituality and sexuality. Both are passionate expressions of intimacy, creativity, and love. Both touch us deeply, and stir us on a visceral level. Sexual intimacy with our partner and spiritual intimacy with our Creator have a great deal in common. Sexual alienation and a sense of body-based shame are common experiences among spiritually wounded people.

Terri was such a person, having grown up in a conservative religious family. She believed that to please God, she was not to have sexual feelings of any kind. These, she had been taught, were "lustful" and "sinful." Rather than learn how to behave in a sexually responsible manner, Terri avoided any possibility of failure by becoming numb to her own body's longing for sexual expression.

Terri had assumed that, once married, she would enjoy sexual intimacy with her husband. So had Carl when he married Terri. Unfortunately, Terri's spiritual wound was extremely profound. Rather than take pleasure in sex, Terri felt ashamed of her body and repulsed by sexual intimacy. Afraid to tell Carl how she really felt, she pretended to enjoy sex with her husband. That's when the migraine headaches began.

Terri's body told the truth, even though Terri tried to hide her authentic feelings. Wounded by religious teaching that divided her from her body, she was unable to fully express love to her husband. Terri's experience is all too common. Many people have been wounded sexually by distorted religious teachings, resulting in a myriad of sexual and relational difficulties including sexually promiscuous behavior, obsession with pornography, diminished sexual desire, impotency, vaginismus, gender confusion, dyspareunia, and other sexual dysfunction.

As spiritually wounded people, we believe that to please God we must deny, hide, avoid, mistrust, and control our sexual feelings. Healing begins when we include our bodies in the spiritual journey.

Cutting Ourselves Off from God

A second way we may respond to spiritual abuse is by developing a distorted view of God. As illustrated in earlier chapters, our early childhood experiences color our ability to give and receive love and nurture. Child abuse and neglect can impair not only our ability to relate to other human beings but our ability to relate to God as well.

Many of us were raised in religious traditions that promoted distorted images of God. Some view God as being abusive which may take the forms of rigid judge, cosmic shamer, or demanding narcissist. Terri, for example, was devout in her faith but actually viewed God as cruel and dangerous. Prior to her marriage, Terri was told that God would be angry with her if she expressed her sexual feelings. In addition, she was promised that God would give her the marriage she dreamed of only if she suppressed her sexuality and remained a "good girl."

Following these instructions to the letter, Terri separated herself from her body and her sexuality. But when the promised "perfect" marriage did not materialize, Terri secretly blamed

God. In fact, in moments of honesty, she realized she hated God for appearing sadistic.

In addition, Terri felt abandoned by God. She cried alone, feeling hopeless that God would or could help her. Like others, Terri related to God as an Absent Parent.[6] Many of us have felt abandoned by God, especially those of us who have experienced any form of abuse whether that be spiritual, physical, sexual, emotional, or neglect. Thoughts go through our minds such as "Where was this so-called loving God when I needed protection and nurturance? How can such a powerless God help me now? If God could help, what makes me think God cares about someone like me?" Losing our faith in a loving Presence, we can feel isolated, unprotected, and alone.

Another variation on "God as Absent Parent" is the God who is thought to be everywhere. Many believe that God is an energy force of nature. On the surface this may have some appeal, but a closer look reveals an underlying spiritual wound that leaves us alone in the universe with no one to care about us.

An energy force lacks the essence of personality which includes the capacity to feel, to choose, or to create. To have a God that is everywhere is actually to have a God that is nowhere. Such a God cannot feel compassion for us and cannot chose to act on our behalf. This God would be unable to create our marvelous bodies through which we could receive spiritual guidance.

Healing comes into our lives when God is experienced as a separate being who interacts with us. But as spiritually wounded people we have difficulty experiencing God as an attentive and loving presence in our lives. Attributing the abusive or abandoning characteristics to God can have a seriously negative impact on us. In the same way that a mother's misattunement to her baby can result in long lasting emotional and physical damage, misattunement between ourselves and God can have serious spiritual ramifications.

Becoming a Body Worshiper

While some may respond to spiritual abuse by "denying the body" and trying to rise above fleshly desire, others respond by worshiping the body. Elevating the body to what may be considered divine status, these people find themselves completely devoted to the maintenance and development of their bodies.

"Fitness fanatics" can be as devout as any other religious addict, committing time, money, and energy to the pursuit of the perfect body. A person may try feel acceptable by carefully sculpting their body into a specific form. An excessive focus on the body cuts a person off from a relaxed sense of acceptance and intimacy with others.

First, a body worshiper tends to work out alone and devote attention strictly to cultivating fitness. In his article, "The Body Politic: Can Fitness Buffs Become a Force for Social Change?", Robert Chianese points out that "concerted group action seems foreign to exercise. While camaraderie may spur one on to more repetitions or laps, rarely does it promote friendship or genuine teamwork." [7]

Rather, excessive exercise requires that fitness seekers develop strict self-discipline. Again, Chianese asserts, "control becomes an end in itself. One must become a control freak to sustain a serious fitness regime . . . One engineers oneself into shape with a calculated narrowness and a dependence on expert authority." [8]

Cut off from intimacy with others and a realistic sense of the limitations of our bodies, a fitness-fanatic views the body as a machine. This body machine is to be crafted into a particular size and shape, and brought under control, rather than to be viewed as a source of information or guidance. The "living essence of the body, its indefinable substance, and its mysterious marriage to self and mind are lost." [9]

Does Your Body Speak of Spiritual Abuse?

What do our bodies tell us about past spiritual experiences? Do our body maps indicate that we suffer from a spirit-body split?

- Each time we pit our heads against our hearts or our spirits against our bodies we illustrate a profound spiritual wound.
- When we take spiritual satisfaction for denying our bodies proper nutrition, exercise, or care we act in accordance with a distorted spiritual perspective.
- Our bodies' reluctance to express sexual intimacy to our partner may indicate an underlying fear of God.
- Headaches, muscle tension, stomach ailments, and other stress-related conditions may speak of anxiety caused by a sense of God's rejection.
- A drive to control the body through excessive exercise and diet illustrate a separation from God and misplaced trust.

Your body map can assist you in determining whether or not you have been negatively impacted by spiritual abuse. The following questions may help you in this endeavor:

1. Attitudes
    » Is my spiritual life a source of comfort or distress for me?
    » Do I feel that I am more spiritual when I reject or deny my sexual feelings?
    » Do I feel that God is abusively demanding? Does it seem like God is absent when I need help?
    » Do I feel driven to have the perfect body?
    » Do I feel loved and accepted by God?
2. Behaviors
    » Do I engage in sexually shaming experiences?
    » Do I try to please God by becoming excessively involved in religious activities?

» Do I spend an inordinate amount of time exercising or caring for my body?

» Do I live a relaxed and balanced lifestyle?

» Do I look to my body for guidance from God?

3. Body sensations

» How does my body feel when I think about God? Does my stomach churn? Does my head ache? Does the stress release from my body and I feel safe?

» Do I rely on my body to guide my exercise program or do I demand that my body give me complete control?

4. Posture

» How do I feel about how I stand? Do I feel proud of my body or ashamed?

» Do I exhibit a relaxed stance, or do I stand hunched over?

5. Breath

» Does my breath denote a sense of acceptance?

» Is my breath shallow or deep? Anxious or at ease?

» What does my breath tell me about my relationship with God?

6. Muscle tension

» Where in my body do I carry tension?

» Does my body illustrate a sense of acceptance, or do I feel I need to do something to prove I am worthy?

» How do the stress points in my body feel when pressed?

» What is God trying to tell me through the tension in my body?

7. Body Memories

» Do I remember feeling loved or judged by God when I was a child?

» Have religious leaders misused their power over me?

» Do images of God frighten or comfort me?

8. Need for Touch

» Do I feel satisfied with the touch I receive from family and friends?

» Do I tend to shy away from people who want to touch me?

» Do I imagine God holding me? Does this image comfort or scare me?

» Has spiritual abuse separated you from your body? Do you include or exclude your body from your spiritual walk? As you trust your body as a means of communication with God, profound healing will come into your life. I invite you to bring your entire self to God so that you can experience complete acceptance and wholeness. Satisfying spiritual intimacy is possible only when love has access to all of you.

Notes

1 Paul Tillich, The Shaking of the Foundations (New York: Scribner's, 1948), 162 (Tillich's emphasis).

2 James B. Nelson, Embodiment: An Approach to Sexuality and Christian Theology, (Minneapolis: Augsburg, 1978), 20.

3 Ibid., 39.

4 Alexander LaBrecque, "To Celebrate the Self" (sermon, Calvary Community Church, Pasadena, California, October 18 1992), 1.

5 Frances Tustin, The Protective Shell in Children and Adults (New York: Karnac Books, 1990), 39.

6 Carmen Renee Berry and Mark Lloyd Taylor, Loving Yourself As Your Neighbor (San Francisco: Harper & Row, 1990).

7 Robert Chianese, "The Body Politic: Can Fitness Buffs Become a Force for Social Change?", Utne Reader, May/June 1992, 69.

8 Ibid., 69.

9 Ibid., 70-71.

Part Three
Your Body Speaks

Chapter Eight

Increasing Intimacy

I anxiously knocked on the door and listened as footsteps approached. The body worker smiled as the door opened, inviting me to follow her to the massage room. After instructing me where to place my clothing, she closed the door behind her to give me privacy.

"What have you gotten yourself into this time?" I chided myself, draping my blouse over the chair. I had called the body worker on the recommendation of my therapist.

"You are a walking head, Carmen," my therapist had said. "It seems like the only purpose you have for your body is to carry your brain around."

"What other purpose could it have?" I smiled at her. Looking down at my body, I had to admit that we were strangers. I was thoroughly cut off from any reason to have a body, except to help me accomplish my various career and intellectual goals. Growing more serious, I challenged, "Look, I came to therapy to deal with my anxiety attacks and depression. What does my body have to do with that?"

"Your body can answer that question for you," was her response. "Your body has a lot to teach you, if you will pay attention."

I didn't want to pay attention to my body. I wanted my body to pay attention to me! After all, I knew what was best. My body was supposed to be my disciplined servant, ready and able to respond to my commands. I expected my body to work long hours without wasting time on sleeping or eating. I had important things to do and needed my body to accomplish my dreams.

And to think my therapist thought my body could actually

teach me something! That notion seemed preposterous. I didn't believe my body had anything to say that I wanted to hear. Whenever my body got my attention, it was always bad news—a pounding headache, a sleepless night, or a stuffy nose. The only time I noticed my body was when it got in the way of something I wanted to do.

"My body's a nuisance," I muttered as I slipped between the sheets covering the massage table. "I don't believe in this massage hocus pocus stuff anyway. What am I doing here? A massage is simply a luxury for the self indulgent. Discipline is what my body needs."

"Are you ready?" the body worker's voice from the hallway interrupted my angry thoughts. Upon hearing I was covered, she entered and asked me to take a long, deep breath. I took a small gasp of air.

"Hmm . . . ," she said, noting my restricted breath. "Let's try that again. Take the breath down into your abdomen." Again I tried to breathe, realizing this breathing business wasn't as easy as it sounded.

"As I proceed, please tell me how the pressure feels to you. And please, concentrate on your breath." Focusing my attention on breathing, I realized that my normal breath was quick and erratic. "I'm breathing like someone who is really scared," I noted to myself.

As I exhaled, the body worker stroked down my back, helping my lungs release the air. She drew her hands up to my shoulders as I took another breath. With her hands, she silently, gently taught me how to breathe more deeply. She urged me to let go, in order to make room for something new and fresh.

I thought to myself, "She is treating my body with more respect than I do." As she synchronized her movements to my breath, the rhythm grew more regular, reaching deeper and deeper into my lungs. A surprising sense of peace and well being slowly replaced my anxiety and irritation.

"Ahhh . . . ," I murmured, relaxing for the first time in weeks, maybe months. "I can take more lessons like this one."

Touch as a Lesson of Love

"Sure," you might be saying to yourself, "this touch business may be easy for you, but this is new and a little scary for me. I've had some difficult experiences in my life that I know hinder my ability to connect with other people. Where can I find someone I can trust?"

I would misrepresent myself if you got the impression that learning how to receive love, especially through touch, has been easy for me. While this journey has been very rewarding, there were times of apprehension. Opening myself up to love is a skill that must be developed over time. It won't happen overnight.

Many approaches to healing are touted these days. "Self help" books sell millions of copies each year in spite of the simple truth that we cannot heal ourselves by ourselves. We just aren't made that way. In the same way we were wounded by each other, we also need each other to heal.

I remember people telling me if I wanted more love in my life, I needed to give more love to others. I suppose the assumption was that I, being too dependent, should appear less needy and offer a better trade to other people. If they wanted what I had to give, they would care for me and give me what I wanted.

I tried that. It didn't work.

I pretended to be independent, a limitless source of care. I gave and gave and gave. What little I had to start with was soon gone. Consequently I found myself worse off than before. I was still feeling the need for more love, only now I was exhausted by my compulsive efforts, resentful over my losses, and depleted of hope.

I now realize I was approaching this problem backwards.

Early infant research shows us clearly that babies who receive love grow into adults who are able to love. Babies who do not receive love, if they survive, grow into adults who cannot love.

I was dependent upon the love of others when I was an infant, and I am still dependent on love. So is everyone else. We all need each other to heal, to expand our capacity to love each other. I believe the goal of adulthood is not independence but interdependence. Happiness is not found in isolation but in beneficial, mutual relationships. As psychologist W.R.D. Fairbairn explains, we do not shift from dependence to independence, but from "infantile dependence" to "mature dependence."[1]

I now have a new definition of love: "To love is to allow another person to make a real difference in one's life, and, because of the difference the other person makes, to act toward the other person so as to assist her or him to develop fully as a person."[2]

The first step in learning how to love others is learning how to *receive* more love, learning to receive care and nurture from others. Like the infant opening her arms to a loving parent, we all need to share ourselves with others in order to grow and to heal. I am finding that as I experience more love, my capacity to love others expands. Loving becomes more like breathing, taking in and giving out, less rooted in my neediness or used manipulatively as a "trade."

The art of loving is learned by sharing love. Unfortunately many of us have been hurt and carry those memories in our bodies. To protect ourselves from further harm, we may push away exactly what we need—the loving and healing touch of another.

Diana was such a woman, afraid to be touched but needing the nurturance terribly. Barely holding back the tears, she came up to me after a workshop. Visibly shaking, she said, "I feel so lonely, so unloved and," her voice cracked, "unlovable. I need more love, but I don't know what to do."

If you are like Diana, wanting more love in your life, I suggest you do something so simple that it may seem almost impossible: open yourself up to more love and nurturance. This recommendation may seem radical, selfish, or foolhardy. In light of past disappointments, isn't it useless to try again? But I urge you to give it a try. All you have to lose is your isolation.

If you, due to the pain of the past, have a pattern of unconsciously pushing away the love that is offered to you, opening yourself to love will require some effort. If you have become touch avoidant because of painful touch in your past, it will take time to change. Like a huge ship turning at sea, the turn won't come quickly as if riding in a speed boat. Grace and patience are required to turn such a magnificent vessel around and head in a new direction. But now you have assistance you didn't know you had before: you have your body map to help you find your way.

Choosing A Traveling Companion

A trip is more enjoyable when a friend comes along to share the fun. Taking a journey, using your body map as a guide, will be more rewarding if you allow others to join you. Selecting a massage or body worker is similar to deciding who you'd like as a traveling companion. After all, it's good to have help figuring out where to turn, especially when traveling in unknown territory.

A massage or body worker can help you read your body map by providing a sense of safety and acceptance. This is created in several ways.

First, we are literally held as our bodies are touched and massaged by the body worker's hands. In our touch-deprived society, many of us long to be held but find that the only avenue available is through sexual involvement. There are times when we need to be held, not as an adult engaged in sexual intimacy, but as a child in need of understanding and nurturance. Like an infant who feels secure in the arms of a loving parent, we can feel "held" by the body worker. This essential need can be met through the nurturing touch of a professional body worker.

Second, we are held through the safe, emotional relationship that develops between us and the body worker. A skilled body worker pays attention to your unique body map, assisting you in identifying information and expressing the feelings your body leads you to explore. Powerful emotions, held captive for years, are respected and explored within the strong walls of the body work relationship or container. You will not be helped if information is uncovered or feelings are released outside of a safe emotional environment and allowed to overwhelm or control you. A skilled body worker can be trusted to share these powerful feelings with you, thereby helping you expand the depth of your healthy relational life.[3]

Kevin, a self-made businessman, came to me for body work because he had recently suffered a mild heart attack. "My doctor recommended I learn how to relax more, so here I am."

As we worked together and Kevin's trust in me grew, a variety of feelings began to surface for him during the sessions. One afternoon I was working on his large, knotted shoulders, and he seemed to melt right into the table. His muscles relaxed significantly, and this ordinarily large man felt small beneath my hands. After the session, Kevin said, "Something new and wonderful happened for me. I felt so safe with you, so accepted. I didn't have to carry the whole world on my shoulders. I knew you were here to share the load." A new level of intimacy developed between us that day.

All of us must feel acceptance from others in order to experience intimacy. This principle is true for all feelings, no matter what kind or intensity—joy, anger, fear, excitement, sadness, longing, safety, happiness. All feelings must be shared in mutually beneficial relationships to bring emotional healing into our lives. "Talking" therapists help us put our feelings into words, using verbal language. Body workers help us share our feelings using the language of our bodies.

Third, an effective body worker becomes what some theorists call a "self-object." A self-object is a person who becomes so significant to us that we actually define ourselves by our relationship to this person. For example, Evelyn, one of my clients, always wore long pants, even in the summer, because she had been told as a child that she had ugly legs. When I touched her thighs, she would often grimace, tighten her leg muscles and clench her hands.

"Am I hurting you?" I asked the first time she did this.

"No," she said sadly. "I'm just thinking how awful it must be for you to touch my legs since they are so ugly."

"Evelyn," I told her quietly, "I can tell you honestly, that thought never came into my mind. I feel honored to be with you, to work with you, and to touch you. I find beauty in your body."

Evelyn began to cry. I continued my work. As the weeks passed and our sessions continued, her physical reaction to my touch grew less severe. Eventually, she stopped flinching altogether. We shared a laugh and a shared sense of accomplishment, when for the first time she showed up for a session in shorts, sporting her "new" legs.

"I realize my legs may look the same to everyone else," she beamed, "but thanks to your acceptance, I now see them with new eyes!"

Everyone needs healthy mirroring from others to help us know how valuable, how lovable we genuinely are. No one ever outgrows the need for this kind of supportive relationship. If we received proper nurture and assurance from relationships during our early years, we will grow into adults who relate freely and warmly with others. However, many of us experienced trauma or deprivation as children and young adults, thereby experiencing "catastrophic loss of self-esteem."[4] To bring healing into our lives, we can now enlist the assistance of skilled body workers to provide us with empathic physical and emotional assurance.

The following guidelines will assist you in locating a trained and qualified massage or body worker who can join you on your journey.

1. Interview Prospective Massage and Body Workers

Since touch has a powerful impact on the body, it is important to select a massage or body worker carefully. I recommend interviewing the worker on the phone when making your first appointment. Feel free to ask about the massage training he or she has received and what type of massage or body work he or she provides. You may want to ask about the theoretical or spiritual approach from which the worker may operate. If you feel comfortable with the phone interview, an appointment can be made. So where can you find a massage or body worker?

Friends and Colleagues: The most reliable route is through personal recommendation. I received the name of my first body worker from the therapist I was seeing at that time. My therapist was acquainted with the body worker's skill and sensitivity. Because I trusted my therapist's opinion and concern for my welfare, I called the body worker and interviewed her on the phone.

If someone you know and trust has a good experience with a massage or body worker, then chances are you may have one as well. This is especially important if you are just beginning to explore massage or body work. Workers come in all sizes, shapes, abilities, and theoretical orientations. It will take time for you to discover which approach is best for you. Maximizing your chance of locating a sensitive and qualified worker will help you have the best possible experience.

Local Massage Schools: Massage schools tend to have qualified instructors who also maintain private practices. Also, students, eager to practice their newly developing skills may be available at a reduced rate. Massage schools are located all over the country to provide training for massage and body work students. Credible massage schools will be certified by the state in which you live. Each state has its own criteria for certification. Your local phone directory or state certification listing may give you the name and phone number of a school in your area. If you have any questions about the calibre of a particular school, I recommend you contact the state for guidelines and certification qualifications.

Established spas, gyms, and hair salons: As massage and body work are growing in popularity, more spas and gyms are hiring qualified workers. A spa or gym, offering legitimate massage and body work services, will be licensed to hire certified workers. Many places I have visited display proper license and certification forms in the reception area or in the massage room. Feel free to ask to see licenses and certification. Decline a massage from any establishment that cannot or will not provide documentation of legitimate status.

While not always the case, spas, gyms, and hair salons tend to hire massage workers rather than body workers. Instead of focusing on inner healing or therapeutic touch, these massage workers usually concentrate on stress management, relaxing after a workout, or self-nurturing experiences. I have thoroughly enjoyed the massage sessions I've received from workers employed at such places, and have, upon occasion, discovered an especially talented body worker in this locale.

Advertisements: I have found some very good massage and body workers through the phone book. I recommend this approach once you've had some experience with massage and body work so that you know what you are looking for. If you are exploring massage and body work for the first time, I do not recommend this route. Deciphering advertisements to find exactly what you want from a session requires time and experience. This route offers you the least amount of information and therefore the most risk of being mismatched. Until you have received a number of massages or body work sessions and are clear about what you really want, I recommend that you take the more reliable path to locating a quality worker, the referral of someone you trust. (For your first sessions, I suggest you start with a worker who comes highly recommended from someone you know or through a reputable spa, massage school, gym, massage clinic, or other establishment.)

2. Select someone you trust

Randy seemed especially relaxed for a first session. His muscles were very receptive to my touch, with large knots releasing with minimal pressure. Usually it took several sessions for a client to feel this comfortable with me, needing to learn first hand that I would protect their safety and dignity in a body work session.

I had nearly completed the session, intending to finish with Randy's right arm. I reached for his wrist and when I lifted it, the entire arm moved as if fused into a solid block of wood.

"Randy, relax your elbow," I said quietly.

Randy, with eyes shut, nodded. Nothing happened. "Randy, relax your elbow," I repeated. Without opening his eyes, Randy said, "I am relaxed!"

I smiled. "Randy, open your eyes and look at your elbow." He opened his eyes and was shocked to find his arm, stiff as a board. "I thought I was relaxed!" We chuckled together.

"What does the tenseness in your arm say to you?" I asked Randy.

"I guess I wasn't willing to give you so much control after all!" he explained. "I was so sure I trusted you, but my arm tells me I intend to let you know who is in charge here. I guess I should make it relax, huh."

"Oh, not at all," I advised. "Let's listen to your arm. It's vitally important for you to feel safe here. I am here to assist you in accomplishing what you want to achieve, not to take your power or take charge. Your arm is telling us both a very important message. You call the shots in this session, from beginning to end."

One of the most important aspects of selecting a worker is finding someone you can trust. Relaxing in a massage or body work session is possible only if you have confidence in your worker to treat you with respect and to work with you in meeting your personal goals. A trustworthy massage or body worker is someone you can rely on to honor your emotional and physical boundaries.

Trust can be difficult if your boundaries have been violated by others in the past. Your body map may remind you of these past hurts through a fast heart rate, muscle tension, agitation, or rapid breath. Rather than discard, excuse, or override these sensations, I recommend that you talk about these issues with your massage or body worker.

You will learn a great deal about someone by the way he or she responds to your body's concerns. An insensitive or untrustworthy body worker will ignore your body's signals to change pace, alter pressure, or take a new direction. If your body's distress signals continue or even increase, you can be certain that this particular massage or body worker is not suited for your needs.

On the other hand, a trustworthy massage or body worker will respect your body and teach you how to more fully honor the messages you receive from your body. Continue only with a worker that inspires trust. Trust will be illustrated by an emotional sense of well being as well as the various clues your body will give you. Each body illustrates trust in unique ways, which may include a slowed pulse rate, deeper breath, relaxed muscle tissue, and/or enjoyment of the touch received.

As you honor your body through touch, your ability to trust will increase. Not only will you enjoy a deeper sense of intimacy with your body worker but also with friends, family, and other people in your life. Your body map will lead you to those who are worthy of your trust, giving you the opportunity to enjoy increased intimacy and nurture.

3. Select a Person Who Is "Attuned" to You

Just as it is important for a parent to attune to the needs of a baby, so it is critical for the massage or body worker to attune to the needs of the client. For healing and growth to occur, you and the worker must share in the experience in such a way that your needs are recognized and addressed.

A positive reaction on the part of the parent "mirrors back to the child a sense of self-worth and value, creating internal self-respect." In much the same way, a massage or body worker can mirror back to us a positive response to our bodies and ourselves. We know that "parental responses of indifference, hostility, or excessive criticism reflect low worth and consequently inhibit the child's assertiveness."[5] Likewise, a mismatched body worker can give us inaccurate and negative feedback about our bodies. It is critical that we select a massage or body worker with whom we share genuine care and affection.

We needn't pursue the "perfect" body worker, however. The goal is to locate a "good enough" caretaker, someone who can provide us with a safe, nurturing, and respectful environment and who will pay attention to our legitimate needs and concerns.

4. Decide If You Want to Work with a Male or Female Massage or Body Worker

As infants, we needed touch from our mothers and our fathers, from men and from women. The gender of our massage or body worker therefore can be important. Personally, I benefit from receiving massage and body work from both male and female workers. Take time to consider which may be most beneficial to you at this time. Some people have very strong preferences, feeling comfortable being touched only by men or only by women. Follow your body's guide in this regard.

I have spoken with some men who are comfortable only if a woman is touching them. The sexual feelings related to massage are such that touch, for them, must be relegated to "heterosexual" interaction. Other men, by contrast, have expressed a need for physical nurture within set boundaries from a male body worker. Often feeling inadequately touched and nurtured by their fathers when they were boys, body work with a male therapist addresses a need that reaches back into their childhood.

Women may have similar concerns. Touch from a male body worker may fill a void left by an inattentive father. Allowing a man to comfort and attend to their bodies' needs for attention can heal long-standing wounds. On the other hand, some women benefit from feminine nurture, providing attention they needed from their mothers. Women touching women can facilitate the healing of feminine wounds and provide needed guidance and insight.

If you are an abuse survivor, you may want to pay special attention to the gender of your body worker. For some, healing is best facilitated when working with someone who is not the same gender as the person who abused you. Feeling free to trust your body worker is of paramount importance. Your body may lead you to someone who in no way reminds you of the abuse you have endured.

On the other hand, some receive more healing by working with someone who is the same gender as the abuse perpetrator. I worked with one woman who was molested by her mother. She was especially fearful of being touched by a woman. We discussed this, exploring if she might be better served by working with a male body worker. After some discussion, she decided that she wanted to work with a woman. She felt that having a woman touch her in a safe, honoring way could help her resolve her deep feelings of mistrust of women. We worked together for over a year, an experience that restored her sense of trust in women and, more importantly, in her own self and womanhood.

Touch can be healing only when your body is honored through out the process. Trust your body, because your body never lies. The direction your body leads you will be undoubtedly the most beneficial path.

5. Develop Additional Support

Holly's stomach turned and her neck muscles tightened as Susan's arm slid around her waist. Even though Holly had known Susan for only a couple of days, having met at a professional conference, the two women had bonded quickly and easily. Susan's touch was the first time Holly had felt uncomfortable with her new friend.

"Are you interested in getting something to eat?" Susan asked, unaware of Holly's discomfort.

Holly realized that in the past she would have ignored her feelings, so as not to make waves. But due to her growing trust of her own body, she decided to try something new.

"Susan," Holly started slowly. "Before we decide on dinner, could we talk here briefly for a moment?"

Susan, a bit bewildered, agreed.

"I value our new friendship and hope that we stay in touch after the conference ends," Holly said.

"So do I," Susan responded in a hopeful way.

Holly took a breath and continued, "And for me to feel safe, I need to be able to tell you when I feel uncomfortable about things."

Susan nodded, "Yes, I want that for me too."

Holly smiled nervously, "Well, I need to tell you that when you put your arm around my waist, I felt uncomfortable."

"Oh, I'm sorry, Holly. I guess I just feel so comfortable with you already, that I acted too familiar with you. I will be more aware of that in the future."

Holly visibly relaxed, "Wow, that was much easier than I thought it would be!"

Susan laughed. "For Pete's sake, woman! I care about you!

I'm glad you told me how you felt. So, what do you say, ready to find some dinner?"

Holly smiled, "I'd love to."

As touch becomes a more reliable source of intimacy within the massage experience, touch becomes more a part of other intimate relationships as well. Because I have received massage and body work from both men and women therapists, I am much more comfortable touching people in general. Rather than feel afraid to express affection through touch, I am more able to embrace my women and men friends with a sense of safety and comfort.

As we honor our bodies, as if by magic, we come into contact with people we can trust, people who will care. Your body will alert you to dangers in relationships you now overlook. Coming close to someone will become safer, as your body gives you needed clues and guidance. As healing comes into your life, I assure you that caring people will be available to you in new and wonderful ways.

If you have decided that body work is the path for you, I strongly recommend that you create a strong support network for yourself. If you are like me, some of the wounds of the past require more attention than friends or family members can give. Consequently, I have effectively utilized professional therapy and self help support groups. I recommend both of these opportunities highly.

The many feelings that surface and the memories that become clearer through body work can be shared with trained therapists and support group members. In much the same way that a mother "attunes" herself to her babies' feelings and thereby makes these experiences a part of intimacy and love, counselors and support group members can attune themselves to us. Each time we talk about what we experienced in a body work session with another person, a deeper healing takes place. When we feel "heard," each time someone "sees" what we're going through, each time another person "feels" what we feel, we are loved. And each time we are loved, we become better lovers.

Honor Your Body

In this and the following chapters, we will go one step at a time, at a pace that is just right for you. I encourage you to pay attention to your body all along the way. Please proceed at your body's rate of comfort, stopping if needed. This brings us to the very important first step: Please make a commitment to yourself now that from this moment on you will treat your body with respect. Your body may not have been treated respectfully in the past. As you read through the first part of this book, you may have identified different ways you have been hurt or deprived. These wounds may affect your ability to protect yourself in the present. Being touch deprived as an infant can cause us to push away positive experiences available now. But just because your body has been denied honor in the past, does not mean that it is too late for you.

I fully believe that today we can all start a new path, no matter what happened to us yesterday. And that new path can and must begin, not when you find the most talented body worker nor after you have had months of massage sessions but right now. Honoring your body starts with you and your commitment to yourself.

Making a conscious commitment to honor your body is so important that, if you are unwilling to do so, I strongly urge you not to proceed with body work or massage. You see, touch is very powerful. It can be the catalyst for healing or untold devastation. The difference between a helping touch and a hurtful touch is the extent to which you and your body are honored by that touch. If you dishonor your body during a massage session, the greatest body worker in the world would not be able to protect you from your own self. Healing starts with you. Honoring your body starts with you. That process can begin now.

I urge you to spend a few moments thinking about the way you have treated your body up to this point.

- Have you paid attention to your body?
- Have you expected your body to pay attention to you?
- Have you treated yourself with respect, or abused and deprived your body of what was needed?
- How do you feel about your body? Are you allies or competitors? Friends or foes?

If you are adventuresome enough, you might actually discuss these questions with your body! You may be surprised to find that you have not treated your body so well, all these years. Most of us have expected our bodies to take care of us, while we complain about how it looks and ignore requests for care. Amy Cunningham, in her article "How I Learned to Love My Body," shares a conversation she had with her body:

> "Hey, I'm mad at you!" my body blurted out.
>
> Given that I was hardly used to hearing my body speak, I surprised myself by having an immediate, if not completely original retort.
>
> "Oh, yeah? What are you mad at me for?" I said. "I'm the one who should be mad at you!"
>
> "Well, first off, you're just not taking care of me," my body said. "You push me until I'm completely spent, then you get mad when I don't look so great."
>
> "Face it," I snapped back. "You'd look like hell even if I didn't push you."
>
> "See? That's what I mean. You basically hate me."[6]

Amy was a brave soul. She was willing to hear what her body had to say. Many of us are not so courageous because we already know we have not honored out bodies. But facing the truth about how we feel about our bodies is a critical step in healthy change.

After making a realistic assessment of your relationship with your body, I invite you to obtain a blank piece of paper, then write out your commitment to yourself. Make a contract with your body, spelling out how you will honor yourself from this day on.

If your experience is similar to mine, you will discover new ways to honor your body as you continue this journey. We all have much to learn about caring appropriately for ourselves. Honoring your body map is a first step, a simple step, a promise to yourself that you will respect your body more than you have in the past. This commitment will deepen as your proceed. Your loving appreciation for your body will expand. It's fine to look forward to growth. It is important now, however, to simply begin.

Notes

1 W.R.D. Fairbairn, "Object Relationships and Dynamic Structure" in An Object Relations Theory of Personality (New York: Basic Books, 1946), 145.

2 Carmen Renee Berry and Mark Lloyd Taylor, Loving Yourself As Your Neighbor: A Recovery Guide for Christians Escaping Burnout & Codependency (San Francisco: Harper & Row, 1990), 64.

3 Frances Tustin, The Protective Shell in Children and Adult (New York: Karnac Books, 1990), 73-74.

4 Howard S. Baker and Margaret N. Baker, "Heinz Kohut's Self Psychology" An Overview, American Journal of Psychiatry 144:1 (January 1987), 2.

5 Ibid., 3

6 Amy Cunningham, "How I Learned to Love My Body," Mademoiselle, April 1992, 100.

Chapter Nine

Increasing Health and Vitality

"My skin is just drinking up the oil, isn't it?" David asked rubbing his arm.

"Yes," I responded, "Your skin seems to be a bit dry and needing some attention."

Closing his eyes and sighing with satisfaction, David said, "Yes, it's true. My skin needs some attention. I need some attention, and this is exactly what the doctor ordered."

Touch can be extremely nurturing, especially in a safe environment where nothing is expected from us in return. Few of us receive the touch we genuinely need. Through massage, our skin is nurtured, which passes on a sense of well being to the other "parts" of ourselves.

What kind of touch experience is best suited for your current needs? How can massage or body work help you read your body map? Which, massage or body work, would contribute most to your present needs for growth and healing?

In order to answer these questions, it is critical to have a realistic idea of what your needs are at this time. Answering the following questions may aid in this endeavor:

1. Do you want assistance handling day-to-day stress?
2. Do you want assistance relaxing sore or tired muscles?
3. Is your focus on the "here and now?"
4. Do you want to simply relax while someone nurtures you?
5. Do you want assistance in dealing with problems from your past?
6. Are you ready to invest, emotionally and financially, in a series of therapeutically beneficial sessions?

7. Do you have a support network in place to help you through the process of dealing with the past?

8. Are you ready to take responsibility for your own inner journey?

9. Is your focus one of integrating the past with the present?

If you answered "yes" to questions #1 – 4, then massage may best suit your current needs. If "yes" was your response to questions #5 – 9, then body work may be more beneficial to you at this time.

"But what's the difference between massage and body work?" you might be asking. The definitions I give here are my own and may not be shared by other massage and body workers you will meet. I have found it helpful to make a distinction between massage and body work in my own journey, as different needs are met by different touch experiences.

In a massage session, the client tends to be fairly passive while the massage therapist takes responsibility for providing a specific service. The focus is primarily on relieving tension held in your body without direct concern about your thoughts, feelings, or interior process. Your mind may wander as the knots in your muscles release, blood and lymph fluids flush out toxins, and your skin is stimulated and caressed.

A massage therapist focuses attention specifically on your body—the elasticity of the skin, the tightness of your muscles, the rhythm of your breath. The primary task of the massage therapist is to relieve muscle tension and to nurture you. That being accomplished, you leave the session satisfied.

Body work, as I use this term, differs from massage in several ways. First, the goal of body work is broader than massage, endeavoring to heal the mind-body-spirit-emotion splits from which so many of us suffer. Touching the body is seen less as an end in itself (as in massage) and more as part of the healing process.

Second, in body work the body is more fully acknowledged as a participant. The various conditions of the body, such as muscle tension, skin sensitivity, and breathing patterns, are considered sources of information—possibly about the past, aspects overlooked in the present, or perhaps guidance for future changes.

Third, the body work client is a relaxed, receptive, yet more active participant than in massage. While your mind may wander as you receive a massage, a helpful body work session requires you to mentally and emotionally join with the body worker to facilitate your healing and growth. Body work is a more disciplined, structured experience than is massage.

Fourth, the body worker usually operates out of a personal theoretical framework that helps you decode and decipher your body map. The body worker focuses on your body as well as your feelings, your spiritual path, your entire well being. The thoughts and focus of attention of the body worker are of immense importance as he or she attunes to your experience.

Both massage and body work have specific benefits. One is not better than the other. I receive both massage and body work sessions on a regular basis and both provide me with unique opportunities for growth and healing.

I rely on massage to help me read my body map's signals regarding the stress of day-to-day life. For example, I have been typing for quite some time now. My arms and hand muscles are tight from repetitive movement. My back and behind are stiff from sitting so long. A massage sounds wonderful to me right now!

I also schedule massage after I return from traveling. Carrying suitcases can strain my arm and back muscles. Sitting for hours in planes, cars and buses can result in muscle tension. We all have regular activities that stress our bodies directly, through strenuous or repetitive motion, or indirectly, through emotional or intellectual stress. Massage can be very helpful to your ongoing functioning and health.

However, to read directions from my body map regarding unexpressed feelings, past experiences, or future decisions, I schedule body work sessions. In the safety of a body work session, I have remembered abusive experiences forgotten by my conscious mind but recorded in my body. Through loving touch, I have grieved losses, released my rage, and opened myself once again to hope and kindness. Confusion has been replaced with clarity, despair with direction.

Because there are many different forms of body work and massage, deciding which best suits your needs can be quite a task. As new body work and massage approaches are continually created and refined, it is easy to become overwhelmed by the choices. Because of the variety available to us today, I will not attempt to describe all the types available to you. I will, however, share with you a couple of guidelines that have proven helpful to me.

When I first started exploring body-oriented healing practices in the mid-1980s, I wanted to "get fixed" as soon as possible. So I signed up for programs that promised to straighten me out (literally) in ten, five, or even one easy session. Well, often I was straightened out—after some of these sessions I even walked differently—but these sessions weren't that "easy." In fact, the workers worked so deeply in the tissue that these sessions were downright painful.

Jules Older explains, "Through the ages practitioners of massage have chosen sides around the issue of pressure. The hardliners maintain that for massage to do any good it must go deep, a position equivalent to the theory that for cough medicine to work it has to taste bad. The other side puts more emphasis on feelings of warmth and pleasure and on the personal contact offered by soothing hands."[1]

I've spoken with many people over the years who claim that the more radical, often painful approaches have helped them tremendously. One man told me he believes deep work, sometimes referred to as "restructuring body work" literally saved his life. After having a serious heart attack, he received restructuring body work which helped him work through a great deal of rage and grief. He believes that this reduction in stress is helping him ward off another heart attack.

Often focused on deeply held feelings and trauma, radical approaches endeavor to restructure the body rapidly. But, if your body's like mine, it isn't going to like it. It's going to hurt.

Not only is radical body work and massage more painful, it is also riskier physically and emotionally. I do not doubt the effectiveness of body restructuring approaches. To the contrary, I am convinced that restructuring body work has the power to produce major changes in the body. I have personally experienced these tremendous changes but also felt emotionally overwhelmed by the pace of movement.

We've all heard the saying, "no pain, no gain." Quite frankly, I think this idea is bogus. It was probably developed by someone who didn't like his or her body very much. I believe that pain is the body's way of saying, "Hey! Knock that off!" A basic message. A sound interpretation.

When in doubt about a specific approach to body work or massage, I look for guidance from babies, who often seem to be wiser than most of the adults I know. Babies don't like pain. Their bodies withdraw from pain and draw them to pleasure. That route is good enough for me.

Over the course of my journey, I have experienced long-lasting healing from the more patient and rhythmic approaches. The body can be trusted to set the pace, providing a natural pace of healing that allows for the time needed to develop new emotional, relational, and spiritual protective skills.

No matter what type of body work you choose, it's important to trust your body. Don't take my word for what might be best for you. Test out different approaches for yourself. You might find the more radical approaches to your liking. Only you can decide what is best for you.

Health Benefits of Massage and Body Work

I chuckled as I walked Patrice to the door. "You don't look like the same person who came in an hour ago."

Patrice smiled, "I don't feel like the same person. I was so frustrated with the traffic, annoyed with my husband, and stressed out about work. It seemed like I just couldn't cope with it all." Putting on her coat with an air of calm confidence, she boasted, "Now I feel like I can handle anything!"

Like Patrice, most of us live stress-filled lives. In fact, stress is an integral and necessary part of being alive. Dr. Hans Selye, former president of the International Association for the Study of Stress and dean of stress theorists, claims that "Stress is good and bad. The good makes us forge ahead against obstacles. The bad makes us sick."[2] Too little stress and we die of boredom. Too much stress and we die of overload.

How does stress reside in your body? For many, stress shows itself through muscle tension, tightness in the tissue that may even draw up into painful knots. Your primary stress spot may be your neck, lower back, between your shoulder blades, the palms of your hands, or, if you are like me, the middle of your calf. Wherever you have a muscle, you can store stress.

Muscle tension, if unrelieved, can lead to more painful or dangerous conditions, such as tension headaches, back problems, or painful cramping. Stress and distress can be "as much a killer as bug poison. [They] can aggravate such conditions as arthritis, cardiovascular and renal disease, allergy, and, so researchers think, even cancer."[3]

Few people complain about not having enough stress in their lives. Most of us are challenged with coping with excessive stress on a daily basis. Massage and body work assist in releasing day-to-day stress that may otherwise be stored in the body. Since I have been receiving regular sessions, my bouts with common-day illnesses, such as colds and flu have decreased dramatically. I believe that my current state of health is due in part to increased attention my body enjoys through massage and body work.

Clients I've worked with have reported similar experiences. One of my clients named Betty suffers from tension headaches. She remarked as a session ended, "My headache is completely gone! I carried that headache around all day long and couldn't shake it." Rubbing the back of her neck, Betty beamed, "This is great! I will definitely remember this next time my head starts to throb."

Many body workers believe that stress and unexpressed emotions can contribute to illness. Milton Trager, the developer of Tragerwork [R](a type of body work that focuses on the gentle rocking movements and rotating limbs) is convinced that "for every physical non-yielding condition there is a psychic counterpart in the unconscious mind, corresponding exactly to the degree of the physical manifestation." He believes that the purpose of his work is to "break up these sensory and mental patterns which inhibit free movement and cause pain and disruption of normal functioning."[4]

I do not assert that body work can "cure" all illnesses. I do believe, however, that body work can assist us in releasing body-based stress that often contributes to disease. By freeing our bodies of pain and tension, our immune system can be stimulated to fight illness in a more powerful manner. Numerous studies have illustrated that nurturing touch can activate and stimulate the immune system. One way this is accomplished is through increased circulation of blood and lymph fluids during massage and body work.

While the heart pumps blood through our veins, no such pump exists to move lymph fluid through our system. Lymph fluid, designed to cleanse our bodies of toxins, moves through our tissue in one of two ways: movement or massage. When we exercise, the heart pumps faster, sending blood and oxygen through our veins at a quicker and more effective rate. Similarly, movement causes the muscles to contract and extend, thereby moving lymph fluid through our tissue. The flow of blood and lymph fluids are extremely important for the health of our cells, maintaining our immune systems and fighting disease. Massage and body work are effective in increasing blood and lymph circulation without the effort! As we relax through massage and body work, our oxygen intake increases, providing our cells with needed nourishment and cleansing.

Ever hear someone say, "I think I'll take a breather?" We tend to equate our taking deep, relaxing breaths to resting and recuperation.Breath work is often used in body work sessions to, among other reasons, help relax us and bring needed oxygen into our bodies.

Even though I receive massage regularly, it still comes as a surprise how tense I can become between sessions. Often, under stress, I start to breathe in a rapid, shallow pace. Even on the massage table, I can continue this gasping pattern, until the massage therapist reminds me gently, "Carmen, remember to breathe deeply and relax." While enjoying the pleasure of massage, you are actually doing something wonderfully healthy for your body.

Limitations of Massage and Body Work

Massage and body work can facilitate healing and growth in your life. Body-oriented healing can accomplish many things for you. But for this approach to healing to be effective, it's important to recognize not only the potential but also the limitations.

One of the reasons body work and massage have come under negative scrutiny, I believe, is partially due to unrealistic claims some have made about them. It is true that massage and body work can relax the body and encourage the flow of blood and lymph fluids, thereby strengthening the effectiveness of the immune system. Body work, however, cannot be expected to "cure" all of your physical ailments.

In fact, if you suffer from certain illnesses or conditions, it is unwise to receive massage or body work. Medical conditions that do not respond well to or are aggravated by massage include:

- arthritis
- inflammation caused by bacterial infection
- bursitis
- any pressure on nerves
- phlebitis
- cellulitis[5]

Please remember this guideline: "Whenever in doubt, don't touch." If you have any reservations, questions, or medical concerns, always contact a medical physician before receiving a massage or body work session.

I believe that, as you attend to your body through touch, your body map will provide you with valuable, maybe even life-saving information about how to best cope with stress in your life. Rather than relentlessly drive your body to excessive productivity, your body map can guide you to a healthier pace of living. Unavoidable stress can be better managed through the nurturing touch of a massage or body worker. I am convinced that health and vitality increase when we attend to ourselves under the wise guidance and direction of our bodies.

Notes

1 Jules Older, Touching Is Healing, (New York: Stein and Day, 1985), 95.

2 Theodore Cooper and Lee Edson, "Stress, Stress, Stress," Across the Board, (September Vol. 16 1979), 10.

3 Ibid., 11.

4 Richard Leviton, "Moving with Milton Trager," East West, January 1988, 58.

5 James Cyriax, "Clinical Applications of Massage," in Massage, Manipulation and Traction, ed. Sidney Licht, (New Haven, CT: YUP, 1960) 122-144.

Chapter Ten

Integrating Your Past with the Present

Throughout the night, I stood beside my grandmother's hospital bed, hoping she would gain consciousness long enough for me to tell her I loved her, one last time. The next morning I wearily drove home and fell into bed for a few hours of sleep. Abruptly, I was awakened as the phone rang, bringing the news that she had passed away. Through the days that followed, while attending funeral services and seeing grieving family members, I kept my emotions fairly controlled, storing sadness between my shoulder blades and suffering from shortness of breath.

A few days later, my weary body sank heavily onto my body worker's massage table. Once I felt the safe hands of the body worker against my back, my lungs let go of the tension and I began to cry.

My body worker didn't say anything to me. She didn't have to. Her hands said all that needed to be said in the way she nurtured and comforted me through my grief. The tears flowed freely and without shame, bringing to the surface the sadness I had stored in my body over the past several days. A cleansing took place that afternoon as my body worker joined me in my grief and honored the love I had for my grandmother.

The memory of any important experience evokes a reaction from us that is both emotional and physical in nature. As I recalled the various events leading up to and following my grandmother's death, I felt feelings of loss and grief. At the same time, I experienced tension in my back muscles and around my lungs.

When my body and my feelings were unified I experienced comfort from my grief.

A sense of unity and peace is available when the touch relationship between you and the worker is used to balance these three components: 1) an accurate memory of a noteworthy past event, 2) an expression of accompanying emotion, and 3) an accurate interpretation and release of the physical manifestation recorded in the body.

When harmony does not occur between these three components, we become disconnected from part of ourselves. For example, we may remember the event but forget the feeling, like my client, Jerry. With a calm voice, Jerry told me about a time when, as a little boy, he hid with his mother in his bedroom closet as his father tore up the house in a drunken rage. When I asked him how he felt about that experience, Jerry shrugged. "Oh, I don't know. It wasn't that big a deal really. After all, it happened a long time ago."

Once Jerry was on the massage table, however, I found huge knots in Jerry's lower back and thigh muscles. He also clenched his jaw tightly shut so the muscles on the side of his face were hard as rocks. His body spoke of his feelings, but he was yet unable to identify and express how he felt emotionally about this terrifying event.

On the other hand, we may experience the feeling but forget the memory, storing the tension in our bodies. Linda told me that she felt a sense of dread each time I began massaging her left arm. "It feels like you're pinning me down, trapping me somehow," she told me during one session. At her suggestion, I continued massaging her arm during each session, as she noted the feeling dread each time it occurred.

One afternoon, she gasped and pulled her arm away. Sitting up quickly, she said, "I remember now! When I was about five, the neighbor boys chased me and pushed me to the ground. They held me down, pinning my left arm underneath me, while they looked down my pants. I was so frightened and angry. I forgot all about that incident until now."

Linda discussed this insight with her talking therapist for several sessions, expressing rage, sadness, grief, and fear. Eventually her feelings subsided and she could remember that hurtful incident with minimal emotional distress. From then on, massage of her left arm no longer triggered a feeling of dread. The massage just felt good to her.

Not only can we cut ourselves off from our feelings or our memories, we can also numb ourselves to bodily sensations or experience excessive pain that is unrelated to recent injury or accident. Numbness, lack of body awareness, or painful sensations can indicate an unresolved experience from our past.

Through nurturing touch, we can accurately read our body maps, thereby giving us valuable clues to those memories we may have forgotten and those feelings we still need to express. Our body maps give us clues of unresolved experiences when 1) we are cut off from bodily sensation, experience numbness in parts of our bodies or suffer from pain or body tension; 2) we have feelings that seem to come out of nowhere or we lack appropriate feeling for experiences we remember; or 3) we have body tension or feelings that are unattached to any specific memory or experience. These three aspects are closely related and sometimes hard to distinguish from each other. For our purposes, however, I will first discuss the importance of accepting our body sensations. Then I will address the importance of accepting our feelings and, finally, the importance of accepting our memories.

Acceptance of Your Body Sensations

When you are touched, what sensations do you feel? This is a very important question, one that I recommend you ask yourself repeatedly throughout your body work sessions. What are the physical feelings you experience? Are the sensations painful or pleasurable?

When we were infants, prior to interference or misattunement, we were very clear about pain and pleasure. Our bodies let us know in no uncertain terms when something hurt or pleased us. All of us knew instinctively, aided by our God-given bodyselves, that pleasurable sensations are to be enjoyed and painful experiences to be avoided.

As adults, we may no longer be as wise as we were as infants. Many of us now confuse pain with pleasure, mistaking one for the other. Due to childhood neglect or abuse, we may no longer associate positive feelings to pleasure. Instead, we feel ashamed of the pleasure we receive, especially if those good sensations come from our bodies. Some of us find more enjoyment in deprivation or pain than in experiences that affirm or nurture us.

Because of our confusion, accurately discerning pain from pleasure may take time and practice for many of us. Here the body worker can have a major healing impact by teaching you how to pay closer attention to your body in order to discern the messages.

I urge you to pay careful attention to the sensations associated with touch. Feelings associated with knots being pressed and massaged tend to fall along a continuum, from numb on one end to pleasurable on the other. I visualize this continuum like this:

NUMB — EXTREMELY PAINFUL — "GOOD" SORE — PLEASURABLE

<————————————————————————————————>

In my own journey and in my work with clients, I've found that some knots, which are often very hard, produce no sensation whatsoever when pressed. Often my client will request that I press hard into the tissue so that they can "feel" it. The lack of sensation, however, is rarely due to an insufficient amount of pressure. Rather, this person is cut off from feeling that part of his or her body.

When I work with someone with "numb knots," I tend to proceed very slowly and respectfully. These hard places often hold deep emotions or memories that have been too painful or overwhelming to face directly. I work slowly to see if the person trusts me enough and is prepared emotionally to deal with the feelings or memories held in this tight, hard place.

One client had two large knots, one on each shoulder, near the base of her neck. Even though the knots were large and very hard, she reported little sensation in them. I commented that they were as hard as metal bolts. She opened her eyes and declared, "Yes, that's what they are. They are bolts that keep my head from floating away!"

At the end of our session, we discussed her "bolts." For years she had felt discounted intellectually. Her family, and especially her husband, belittled her intellectual abilities. Now, in her middle thirties, she was in graduate school, pursuing her educational interests, finally strong enough to cultivate her own thoughts and ideas. She told me, "I need these bolts right now. I believe they are my body's way of illustrating my fight to keep my head and my heart together."

Over the next year we worked together, her bolts diminished some but did not fully disappear. Perhaps these knots may eventually relax, but it was important for us to honor these "bolts." She received more from her session because we honored her struggle to integrate her emotional and intellectual development than if we had viewed these knots as "bad," something to reject.

In other instances, a person is ready to release tension. This release may be gradual or sudden. Often there will be a deep soreness that remains in the tissue surrounding that area after the release. Some clients have told me the soreness has lasted a day or two after the session and triggered an emotional reaction such as

sadness, rage, loss, relaxation, or even a deep sense of contentment.

If the knot does not release after some loving attention, I
gently massage the area. But I do not insist that the knot release. I
follow the body's lead, and work with the person to build a sense
of trust and safety, so that perhaps during our next session together, the knot will release.

Sometimes the knot will not release, but the numbness is
replaced by extreme pain. Honor genuine pain, especially sharp
or piercing pain, as a warning sign to slow down or go in a different direction. Once during a session when I was the client, I
ignored the pain in my own body and did not tell the body
worker of the pain's severity. Thinking that I was comfortable, the
body worker pressed deeply into my leg muscles. The next morning I woke up with six large, dark bruises on my calf and thigh
muscles. Because I had ignored my body's signals, I suffered tissue damage, a visual reminder of how poorly I cared for my own
body.

The most helpful sensation to experience while having a knot
pressed is what I call that "good sore" feeling. The knot is soft
enough to allow blood and lymph fluid to move through the
tissue, bringing oxygen and nutrients to the area. Often a sense of
relaxation flows through the body, as these knots begin to release
their hold. Taking a deep breath, clients often sigh out loud, visibly relaxing their entire bodies, not merely the small area containing the knot. It is common to simultaneously experience
emotion moving through the body as well.

When an area is free of tension, the most common experience is one of pleasure. A gentle massage nurtures tissue, drawing
blood and lymph fluid through the area. Feelings most often
evoked are happiness, contentedness, safety, and well being.

Acceptance of Feelings

In addition to paying attention to body sensations, it is important to experience the emotions that are connected to the body. Ask yourself "feeling" questions throughout the body work session. These might include:

- What feelings does the tightness in my right calf trigger?
- When I breathe more regularly and deeply, what emotions fill my chest?
- When my feet tingle during a massage, what feelings are being released?
- Do I feel sad or angry when the knots between my shoulder blades are pressed?
- Does the tightness in my thighs signal distress or rage, determination or defeat?
- When my scalp is massaged, do I relax or tense up?
- Are my neck muscles open to touch, or do they fight back in defiance?

In body work, we have the chance to share feelings, some for the first time, with someone who is able and willing to be with us through this powerfully healing journey. Since we may consider some of these feelings "negative," we might find ourselves frightened, easily overwhelmed, and unfamiliar with these particular emotions. In fact, these feelings are quite normal and acceptable. But to us they are not because, in our families, these particular feelings were threatening and therefore banned from being shared with others. These feelings may include fear, sadness, sexual arousal, or anger, which are the emotions most commonly experienced in body work sessions.

Fear

"I know I need help," Marjorie told me, "but every time I even think of having a massage, I get sick to my stomach with fear."

I smiled and responded, "Then let's start with what feels comfortable for you. Is there part of your body you would like to have massaged?"

Marjorie looked surprised, "You mean, I don't have to do it a certain way? You will actually go at my pace?"

"Certainly," I said. "Your body is our guide. You are in complete control. Let's take this one step at a time and honor your fear."

Fear is a feeling many of us have hidden in our bodies. Consequently, when we are faced with the possibility of being touched, we may experience an ill defined sense of danger. Often held in our muscles as a memory of past trauma, fear can be carried in our arms, legs, chest, neck, fingers, feet or other parts of our bodies.

Sometimes we fear the experience of touch itself, distrusting anyone who reaches out in our direction. While some are cut off from feelings, others may fear being overwhelmed by emotion. Touching can take on a magical significance, seeming to have more power than it actually has. If you are overly vulnerable to the experience of touch, you may feel insufficiently insulated from the invasion of another person's influence. Forcing yourself to be touched when your body is communicating fear will not bring healing. In fact, such an experience can cause more emotional and physical damage.

If you feel frightened of touch, I urge you to honor this feeling. Perhaps a good place to start is setting up an appointment with a body worker for the purpose of *talking about* touch. There is no law that says you must experience body work in a particular manner. Start where you and your body need to start. A next step may be receiving a five-minute foot, hand, or neck massage. For example, I've benefited greatly from having a body worker concentrate on my feet when I am feeling fearful. A foot massage tends to strengthen my feelings of safety and competence, giving me a sense of "grounding." You may have other areas of your body more open to touch than others. Perhaps this approach will help you release your fear. Allow your own body to guide you through the anxiety and fear.

As you feel comfortable, you can increase the length of the massage or add new areas of the body. Take it one step at a time, following your body's lead. Your fear is with you for a reason, and following your body's lead will naturally bring you to a point of healing.

Sadness

While I was attending to Dale's calf muscles, he sighed deeply and woefully. I asked, "Are you experiencing a particular feeling right now?

"Yes," he said quietly, "Your touch on my knee reminded me of when I was injured in a football game, back in high school. That was it for me. In an instant, my dream of being a pro snapped with my knee. Maybe it was just a foolish, boyhood dream, but I guess I'm still sad about it. I hardly ever think of it now. Funny how this session brings all that back to me."

Body work can provide us a safe place to release pent up grief and sadness. Often afraid to cry in front of others, we "swallow" our tears, hold our breath, and keep ourselves from showing our pain. Releasing these feelings of sadness and loss can result in various forms of physical expression, including crying, deeper breath patterns, muscle shaking or coughing. We can utilize body work sessions to share feelings we may be reluctant to share any-where else.

Sexual Arousal

Hank sat in the chair with one leg locked around the other, his arms adamantly crossed over his chest. He looked like a for-tress with the drawbridge clamped firmly shut or a circle of cov-ered wagons heavily armed, awaiting attack. Eyeing me with suspicion, but with a trace of a smile on his lips, he asked provocatively, "I want a massage, but I feel funny about taking my clothes off." He smiled seductively, "Aren't you afraid of the vice squad?"

Hank's reaction to massage is quite common. Many of us equate touch with sex. It may be hard to imagine being touched by another adult without also imagining a sexual encounter. For Hank, receiving a massage meant having sex with someone other than his wife. The prospect of being sexual with someone other than a monogamous partner can trigger a variety of feelings such as anxiety, desire, fear, passion or guilt. Since Hank tended to eroticize all forms of touch, he was conflicted about receiving a body work session.

"It feels odd," he told me, "having you touch me. It's not just about my marriage. It's about my relationship with God. My spiritual life is very important to me, and I feel guilty about having someone touch me other than my spouse."

As we discussed previously, spirituality and sexuality are closely linked within our psyches as fundamental elements of our identity. We often define ourselves in terms of our spirituality and sexuality. I believe that we cannot separate our spirituality from our sexuality without tragically violating our very essence. We are at our core spiritual, sexual beings. If we engage in sexual activity that violates our spirit, we damage ourselves in profound ways. Conversely, if we dedicate ourselves to spiritual practices that deny our sexuality, we also violate the person God meant us to be.

If we truly honor our spiritual selves, embracing our potential to wholeness, we will find ourselves honoring our sexuality as well. And as we honor our sexual selves, we will also honor our spirit. One aspect of our being cannot be truly honored without honoring the other.

Body work can confront us with our spiritual and sexual woundedness. Like Hank, many of us have eroticized touch to such an extent that we cannot imagine touch without being sexually stimulated. However, even the most satisfying sex life cannot meet all of our needs for touch and affirmation. By overly eroticizing touch, we deprive ourselves of experiences of love and nurturance that we desperately need.

If touch triggers a sense of shame or sexual embarrassment for you, as with any other body-based emotion, I urge you to follow your body's lead. As with fear, I recommend that you begin slowly, perhaps with a talking session as a first step. Reclaiming your body for the nurturing experience of touch can take time.

We may be afraid of sexual feelings overpowering us or making us vulnerable to inappropriate sexual contact, or we may resist feeling sexual out of fear of rejection or ridicule. These feelings are most common for those of us who have been sexually violated or spiritually abused and thereby separated from our wholesome sexual selves. Experiencing full acceptance of our sexual feelings can bring needed healing to our spiritual and sexual wounds.

Body work gives us the chance to experience all kinds of feelings, even sexual ones, in a safe environment with someone we can trust. A skilled and ethical body worker will provide strong, safe boundaries to contain sexual feelings. While it is common for sexual feelings to be triggered in a body work session, at no time is it appropriate for a body work or massage session to become a sexual encounter. The body worker is responsible for setting clear sexual boundaries and providing you with a safe place to feel all of your feelings.

As a guideline, remember that you are to be covered with proper draping (sheets, towels, or clothing) at all times, with only the part of the body that is being worked on exposed. At no time are your genitals to be touched. Other areas of your body are to be nurtured but not sexually stimulated.

Should your body worker violate your sexual boundaries, speak up immediately and inform him or her of your feelings. Most will immediately respond by apologizing and negotiating proper boundaries. If this is not the case, terminate the session immediately.

Sexual feelings may be triggered through appropriate, nurturing touch. These feelings are quite normal. It is common to long for deeper intimacy with someone who is nurturing and accepting. If you should feel sexually aroused in a body work session, I recommend that you discuss these feelings with your body worker. A skilled body worker will honor your sexual feelings, while maintaining proper boundaries. As with talking therapists and other professional caregivers, sexual feelings are to be acknowledged but contained.

Anger

The knot was painful, buried beneath Fletcher's shoulder blade. "Ow!" he complained as I pressed into the hard mass. "I want you to dig that out of there," he gasped between clenched teeth.

Decreasing the pressure, I asked him to visualize the knot. After a few moments of silence, he told me the knot was a small "cherry bomb," about to explode. As I worked on the knot, he began to talk about his angry feelings toward his fiancee, his mother, and other women who he felt had hurt him.

Anger is a feeling that frightens many of us. We are often concerned that, if we feel the depth of our anger, we will hurt other people. Again, I stress that it is important to learn how to FEEL feelings without being compelled to act these feelings out in damaging ways. Body work can help us learn this valuable lesson. Too often people who are recovering from child abuse or deprivation get mired in their rage. As Heidi Vanderbilt, in her article Incest: A Chilling Report, explains "Anger feels so good, so powerful, that it can be mistaken for health. Victims, who have often long denied their feelings, need to have their anger and to move through it into healing. From anger springs the energy that propels survivors out of the victimization and into life." But the anger must be focused in appropriate ways, or it can become "all-consuming, all-encompassing. You can drown in it. Anger isn't the last stop, it isn't the goal."[1]

Often we use our bodies to carry anger, because we do not know how to feel angry without hurting someone or ourselves. This may illustrate a breakdown in our relationships with our parents, dating back to our infancy. We can learn how to appropriately feel and express anger by allowing our bodies to release the anger we have stored up over the years.

Anger is stored in many ways. A favorite of mine is between my shoulder blades. Some say that our arms and hands naturally clench when we are angry as a physical preparation to hit our assailant. If we do not follow through with the blow (and rarely is physical violence appropriate), then we store the tension in our arms, specifically in the muscles between our shoulder blades. As we learn to feel anger and channel that energy into making the changes needed in our lives, our bodies can release this self-damaging emotion.

We open ourselves up to emotional healing by sharing our true feelings with another caring, loving human being. All of our feelings are good and wholesome. Just because we feel an emotion does not obligate us to act out this feeling in any particular way. As adults, we can learn how to express our feelings in a variety of ways. Your body worker can help you feel feelings you may never have been able to share before. Then, within the safety of the body work container, you can learn how to express these feelings in helpful, loving ways.

As we learn how to share these feelings, it may be helpful to include your talking therapist, support group, and friends in the process. The more people with whom you can share new feelings the better. Plus, you will have the benefit of many ideas on how to best express these new emotions in ways that enhance rather than damage your relationships.

All kinds of feelings can be shared in a body work session—

love, grief, anger, confusion, terror, loneliness, frustration, satis-
faction.Body work is a healing experience within the context of a
relationship between you and the body worker. A body worker
can provide what you may not have received as an infant: affect
attunement.

As discussed previously, we are able to experience and express only those feelings that have been previously shared with
others. Feelings that have been rejected by others remain cut off
from ourselves and our relationships. By paying attention to your
body and sharing the feelings you experience during the session,
your body worker can help repair damage caused in infancy, early
childhood, and other times in your life.

Affect attunement also results in an increased ability to self
regulate your feelings outside the session. As the body worker
comforts us, we can learn how to better comfort ourselves. As we
are soothed, we can become more adept at calming ourselves. We
do not become dependent upon the body worker in a negative
sense, forever tied to a particular person. Rather, as we are allow
ourselves to be vulnerable to this form of nurturance, we move
beyond infantile dependency and become adept at mutually dependence with those we love.

Acceptance of Memories

If we have consciously forgotten the horrible things that have
happened to us in the past, why think about them now? Why not
leave the past in the past and go on? Why remember?

Many of us carry the pain of the past in our bodies. We are
afraid to be touched, reluctant to re-experience the sadness, fear,
hurt and confusion. But holding in the pain will not free us of its
sting. Turning away from touch will not keep us safe. Only when
we open ourselves and our bodies, once again, to the nurturing

power of touch can we be free, once and for all, from the pain of the past.

There are many benefits for retrieving body memories. A past event that has been successfully resolved is one that we can chose to remember at will. While some of the specific details of the event may have become fuzzy, we are able to retrieve the memory and remember feelings we may have had without undue distress in the present. For example, I remember falling down an embankment when I was ten years old. At the time, I was terrified and suffered cuts and bruises from the fall. Even though I can remember the feelings I had during the experience, recalling that afternoon no longer triggers those feelings. That scary experience does not keep me from skiing or participating in other activities in which I might find myself in a similar place. I learned from my mistakes that afternoon and now live with the memory and the valuable lessons. All three aspects are in line: 1) I am able to remember the experience clearly; 2) I can recall my feelings accurately; and 3) my body has released the pain of the trauma.

Experiences that are not resolved may be hidden from our conscious memories, often exerting an unseen power over our current lives. Unremembered traumatic experiences often limit our choices and trigger feelings that seem confusing to our conscious minds. If we are able to remember unresolved experiences, we often feel all the same feelings we did when we were actually going through the experience. Sometimes referred to as a "flashback," this kind of experience is a "memory without distance. It can bring all the terror of an original event, triggered by something utterly innocuous."[2]

Remembering undigested experiences frees us from being haunted by "inexplicable and confusing emotions, symptoms, and behaviors, with a resultant decrease in feelings of 'craziness' and self-hatred."[3] This allows us to arrive at a realistic rather than idealistic assessment of one's family and one's childhood.

Survivors of deprivation and abuse often suffer from low self esteem. "In a sense, the survivor's body, or at least the survivor's comfort and ease in his or her body was stolen. Since the body was integral to the trauma, it must be integrated into the healing process." [4] Memory resolution allows us to retrieve and integrate "the fragmented aspects of the self, isolated affects, and split off events, resulting in a reversal of the dissociative process and increased feelings of wholeness." [5] As an accurate picture emerges of past abuse, with responsibility placed appropriately on the offender, a sense of personal worth and respect often grows. We come to value ourselves more highly when we realize how much we have overcome successfully.

A word of caution is in order here, aptly expressed by therapist Dr. Elaine Westerlund. "With these benefits in mind, the process of uncovering and validating memories may be cautiously approached. The survivor must have sufficient professional and personal support to carry out the work, the survivor's pace must be continuously monitored, and the risks in terms of functioning must always be carefully assessed." [6] With the appropriate support and respect for the challenges of memory retrieval and resolution, we can work with our bodies toward healing and growth.

What Is a Body Memory?

A body memory is a recollection of a past event that has been stored in the body. Westerlund explains, "Most people assume that a 'memory' will automatically include a visual component. While this may be true for nontraumatic events, it is often not the case with trauma memories due to the role of dissociation and repression." [7] Traumatic or extraordinary events are experienced through all of our senses, body memories are not limited to visual recollections. The sounds, smells, tastes, and physical sensations experienced during the event are stored in the body along with the visual memory.[8] These include:

- Sounds: Auditory memories involve the sounds that were heard during the experience such as the sounds of yelling, crying, breaking of objects, crashing thunder and falling rain, or even an eerie silence. Some people report hearing phrases inside their heads such as "If you tell I'll hurt your parents!", "Please leave me alone!", or "You stupid kid. Can't you do anything right?"

- Smells: During the retrieval of a body memory, you might smell similar odors or fragrances that were present at the time of the event. These smells may include the cologne or body odor of someone who hurt you, gas fumes of a car accident, or the medicine odors of the hospital surgery room.

- Tastes: A distressing experience may have included a variety of tastes such as blood from a beating, semen from sexual abuse, or food eaten prior to a bout of illness.

- Physical sensations: Your body often remembers how you were touched during a difficult experience. For example, you might feel the sting of a belt across your back, the weight of a pillow pressed against your face, or the grip of a hand grabbing your wrists. Physical sensations can be experienced in any part of your body and range from soft, tingling feelings to sharp, distressing pain.

Dr. Westerlund explains that, "Visual memories, when they occur, generally do so as a serious of image 'stills' which must be pieced together over time. Images may be accompanied by a range of sensation and feeling from very little to extreme, partly depending upon the survivor's defenses. Some survivors experience visual memories which are more 'movie-like' through dissociative episodes referred to as flashbacks. During such episodes the abuse is often re-lived as if occurring in the present."[9]

A memory may be triggered through touch. This may occur when: 1) the touch is reminiscent of the actual event, or 2) a memory is being held symbolically and is then released when massaged.

Literal Memories

Memories that are carried in the body can surface through "present life circumstances or situations which are somehow reminiscent of the past. For example, a bodily injury or medical procedure may put a survivor in touch with familiar feelings of physical pain accompanied by helplessness and fear. Or weight loss may heighten body awareness, calling up familiar feelings of self-consciousness and physical vulnerability."[10]

Circumstances or situations that trigger memories may include facing surgery, engaging in sexual intimacy, visiting the scene of the abuse, experiencing a car or other accident involving physical injury, becoming pregnant, seeing a film or television show depicting a similar experience, or meeting someone with similar characteristics of someone who hurt you.

Sometimes memories are triggered through touch, as the body worker massages a part of the body that endured trauma. For example, during my training, I worked with another student as we learned how to massage the feet and ankles. As I worked on her ankles, she had a visual memory of having a brace on her legs as a small child. She told me that she had no conscious memory of wearing a leg brace, but would call her mother right after class to ask.

At our next class, she told me that her mother had confirmed her suspicion. In fact, as a toddler had been diagnosed with a medical problem that called for a painful brace to be worn at night. Her mother told her that, as a little girl, she would cry herself to sleep at night because of the pain. This memory had been kept in her body, but out of her conscious memory, locked away until she had felt the safety of our massage class and the nurture of my hands on her ankles.

Symbolic Memories

Dan carried a large knot in his bicep, that usually felt numb when I pressed it. In this particular session, however, he yelped in pain when I worked on his arm.

"Wow," he commented in surprise, "That is painful."

"I'll take it slower," I responded. I worked lightly on his arm, soothing the sore area. I suspected from Dan's expression that a memory or feeling was coming up for him. After a few minutes, I asked him to share his experience.

He told me, "In my mind, I heard my dad's voice say, 'You good for nothing, wimp. How'd I ever get a weakling like you for a son.' " He paused, "I had forgotten he use to say that to me. I wonder if that's why I work out so hard these days. Trying to build up my arms so I'll be seen as a strong man."

While Dan had never been hit on the arm, his bicep came to symbolize his strength, his manhood, his acceptability. And that is where Dan's body map chose to store that particular emotional wound.

Dan's experience is quite common. Most of us symbolize our pain, our losses, our shame within our bodies. Our challenge is to pay attention and sort through the possible interpretations, until we can properly decode what our bodies are trying to say.

How to Retrieve Memories

Touch can assist in retrieving unintegrated memories. As Timms and Connors point out in Embodying Healing, "The bodyworker's touch must not and does not duplicate the original traumatic touch, nor does it need to. No *reputable* bodyworker (or psychotherapist) would ever touch or stimulate the genital area of a client."[11] Nor would a qualified body worker inflict any other type of abuse such as physical, spiritual, or emotional abuse on a client.

Abusive touch is unethical. Fortunately, it is also unnecessary because "traumatic memory is stored with emotion-linked chemicals in the body and the brain . . . The bodyworker's touch may stimulate similar emotions that re-release these messenger molecules, thus allowing a previously repressed memory accompanying that feeling to arise in the client's conscious memory."[12]

Pay attention to physical sensations you have during or after a body work session. Do you find that some areas of your body are especially numb? especially sensitive? What areas of your body are you reluctant to have touched? What areas feel especially good? Interact with your body's sensations using visualization or inner dialogue techniques, asking for specific guidance about past events.

In addition to touch, memories can be invited to surface by stimulating the sense of hearing. Different types of music or sounds can be used during the body work session that may relate to themes of childhood abuse. Often body workers use soothing sounds to help clients relax. Within a sense of safety, sometimes memories will surface.

Two Warning Signals

A skilled body worker will help you pace yourself. Two warnings will signal you if you move too quickly into the realm of emotional expression.

1. "Reliving" the Abuse

Retrieving body memories is a process to be taken seriously and with the help of a network of support. I strongly recommend that, in addition to a skilled body worker, you enlist the assistance of a well-trained talking therapist as well as regular support from a self help or therapy group. Your experiences have been locked away for good reason. They will undoubtedly evoke feelings and present you with challenges that will take time and courage to face.

Both unskilled body workers and unskilled talking therapists have made similar mistakes with survivors of trauma and neglect. You have probably heard of people who have been in therapy or support groups for an extended time, talking about their childhood abuse or rape experiences without any noticeable improvement. Often people "relive" their past abuses during these sessions. Unfortunately reliving abuse does not produce healing. To the contrary, the mind and body experience the reliving of the abuse as another abusive episode. This may actually do more harm than if the person never tried to face the pain at all.

A skilled body worker or skilled talking therapist, in contrast, will assist you in recalling the episode in such a way that you do not relive the abuse. Rather, by using the body, especially the breath, you can be assisted in staying in the present while doing battle with opponents from the past. Proper utilization of the body, can keep us in the present and able to use the many resources available to us now. We were abused in the past because we were overpowered or dependent upon untrustworthy caretakers. Now, assisted by trustworthy caretakers in the present, we can work with our bodies to bring about needed healing.

Again, I stress that you honor your body through this process, setting a pace in line with your body's rhythm. This may take longer than you desire. Therapist Richard Schwartz wisely advises not to rush this process. "It takes as long as it takes . . . internal systems have their own pace. Therapy should be as brief as possible . . . but not briefer."[13]

An unskilled body worker will try to get all of your knots to relax at once. I urge you to terminate a body work session with a massage or body worker who is more concerned about getting rid of your knots than following the pace your body sets. Some knots require time and care as they release. Bodies forced to change overnight may flood a person with overwhelming feelings.

2. Dissociating

If you become overwhelmed or overloaded by a session, you might respond to excessive and frightening emotion by dissociating from the body. "Dissociation, the sense of leaving one's body, can be a strong protection by allowing the survivor to separate from the immediacy of a painful emotional or physical memory of feeling confused, spaced out, or numb."[14] Pay attention if it feels like you:

- space out
- numb out
- split
- float off
- fly away
- lose touch
- go dead
- blur over
- stop time
- switch
- lose track.[15]

Dissociation is a way to cope with overwhelming feelings or experiences. If you are dissociating, the body work session is no longer a safe place for you. It is critical that you inform your body worker that you are separating from the present and from your body. Your body worker and you can retrace your steps to see what frightened or overwhelmed you.

As your body worker synchronizes to the natural rhythm of your body's pace, he or she will help you "become re-associated with bodily and emotional experiences and reclaim forgotten or denied parts of the self and of life. This re-association leads to greater integration of experience with the self, and thus to more complete healing."[16] As a consequence of re-associating your past with your present, you will learn how to soothe and care for yourself with respect and patience. Your body worker will illustrate how you can comfort yourself, read your body's signs of distress or pleasure, and increase your self-soothing skills. These skills can be used outside the body work session and may include relaxation and breathing techniques, rocking and holding self by putting your arms around your body, and self comforting through imagery and visualization.

Learning to Be a "Good Enough" Client

Many of us have learned from infancy to hide emotions we view as unacceptable. We are so good at this that we may even hide our genuine feelings from ourselves. Because the relationship between the client and body worker is mutual, we may unconsciously try to protect our body worker from any feeling we fear may upset or overwhelm him or her.

Therefore be on the alert for accommodating behavior. You may try to be the "perfect" client, trying to conjure up whatever feelings or experiences you suspect your body worker would want you to have. Your healing is possible in the real world, not a perfect one. In the real world, good enough body workers help good enough clients. For you to grow, it is important that the relationship between you and your body worker be emotionally authentic, not "perfect." A skilled body worker knows that all of the client's needs cannot be met and, in fact, not all of the client's needs should be met.

It takes courage and patience to honor feelings, to determine and understand how important they are in the overall scheme of life. Adding the "body dimension" to that task requires even more courage, especially in a society that devalues feelings and the body. Give yourself time. This is not a quick process. All of us have to find our way at the pace of our own individual feelings and bodies.

A Word about Dreams

As you engage in a body work session, stay alert to representations in your dreams. At times, dream images may symbolize abuse or deprivation and may be communicated to you through specific characters or events. At other times, the images may be more accurately interpreted literally as memories. This is more likely to be true when abuse is explicit, involving one or more family members. Therapist Constance Lillas asserts that nightmares "often occur in post-traumatic situations, where reoccurring dreams are actually memories being played over and over in the mind."[17] Particularly terrifying dreams may be, in fact, accurate accounts of a past traumatizing experience.

Also, it may be helpful to pay attention to the ways your body is depicted in your dreams. Are you in your body or floating above it? Is your body the age you are now, or is your body represented at a younger age? What color is your hair in the dream? Is your body bigger than life or smaller or the same size? Often your dreams will tell you valuable information about your body, and what messages your body is carrying.

Your Body Never Lies

Retrieving body memories requires that you trust your own body and the guidance of your body worker. Often we would prefer to believe we are crazy and these awful things did not actually occur, than to believe the truth our bodies convey. I have experienced this firsthand, as I have worked with clients uncovering painful past experiences, and, more personally, as I have come to face my own past.

Perhaps the most painful body memory I have confronted was realizing that I was sexually molested as a toddler. Working with Carolyn J. Braddock, a highly skilled body worker and the author of Body Voices, I experienced what I consider a "full body memory." I could see the woman standing over my crib, watching the light dim to blackness as she stuffed a pillow over my face. I could hear my own cries and frightened panting as I struggled to breathe. Tingling ran up my legs and through my pelvis area as I remembered her fondling me. I also remembered someone suddenly coming into the room as this abusive woman abruptly removed the pillow, acting like nothing amiss was occurring.

All of my senses were involved in this memory, and yet I left the session telling myself it couldn't be true. Fortunately, I had the support of a quality talking therapist and support network with whom I could talk about this experience. The body worker, along with the other loving people in my life, gave me the emotional safety I needed to believe my body. And because my body told me the truth, I was finally able to release this terrifying experience. As my feelings of pain, anger, terror, outrage and confusion were shared by others, healing occurred. Now I can remember this episode without repressing it or reliving it. I recall the horror but feel proud of myself for facing this abuse. And I feel securely loved by those who have shared this healing path along with me.

If you have painful memories to face, expect yourself to doubt your body. You may find yourself saying things like I said to myself such as "I'm out of my mind," "There is no way this could possibly be true," or "No sane person would believe this."

Dr. Westerlund explains, "Because the wish to disbelieve what is becoming more apparent is so strong, the survivor will need to have others hold the belief when s/he is unable and gently confront the self-doubts as they come up."[18] Allow your body worker to hold a belief in your body when you cannot. All of us are dependent upon the care and strength of others when we are forging new ground. As you learn to accurately interpret your body's messages, you will regain your footing, and genuine healing will result.

Embrace the Healing

Tears streamed down the sides of Pam's face as she laid on the massage table. "My sisters used to poke me, tease me about my breasts, pinch me until I was bruised. But you are so kind, so soothing. No one has ever touched me in such a caring way. It feels like you are smoothing away all those past hurts and bruises."

The kind, honoring touch of a body worker can help heal painful memories of the past. A body work session actively engages all parts of ourselves—our conscious and unconscious minds, our spirits, our memories, our feelings. By involving all of ourselves, the wounds and splits from the past can be healed.

The specific area of healing depends, of course, on your particular area of woundedness. For those of us who have been touch deprived, the challenge of body work may be learning to receive nurturing touch. That in itself may be difficult, and yet offer immense healing of past pain. Others may have been physically, sexually, spiritually, or emotionally abused. Retrieving and resolving these experiences may evoke a myriad of emotions, trigger forgotten memories and provide opportunity for resolution.

Notes

1 Heidi Vanderbilt, "Incest A Chilling Report," Lear's Magazine, February 1992, 25.

2 Ibid., 55.

3 Elaine Westerlund, "Memory Retrieval, Management, and Validation in Incest Survivors" (Cambridge, MA: Impact Resources, Inc. 1988), 6.

4 Robert Timms and Patrick Connors, Embodying Healing: Integrating Bodywork and Psychotherapy in Recovery from Childhood Sexual Abuse, (VT: The Safer Society Press, 1992), 13.

5 Westerlund, Memory Retrieval , 7.

6 Ibid., 6,7.

7 Ibid., 2.

8 E. W. L. Smith, The Body in Psychotherapy, (NC: McFarland, 1985), 45.

9 Westerlund, Memory Retrieval , 3.

10 Ibid., 1,2.

11 Timms, Embodying Healing, 31.

12 Ibid., 31.

13 Richard Schwartz, "Rescuing the Exiles," Networker, May/June 1992, 37.

14 Timms, Embodying Healing , 11.

15 Westerlund, Memory Retrieval, 4.

16 Timms, Embodying Healing, 30.

17 Constance Maria Lillas, Alexithymia: Etiology and Treatment Implications for Psychoanalysis (Ph.D. diss., Newport Psychoanalytic Institute, 1992), 39.

18 Westerlund, Memory Retrieval , 4.

Chapter Eleven

Trusting Your Body

I walked into the body work session and the body worker took one look at me and said, "Look at the way you hunch your shoulders! You obviously have had your heart broken so you try to protect your emotions through your posture."

The next week, I was out of town and visited a different body worker. While working on my shoulders, hunched as usual, she said, "I can tell from your posture that you are excessively responsible. Your shoulders sag because you are carrying a heavy emotional load on your shoulders."

Not much later, I was receiving a massage from a third body worker. He informed me that my hunched posture was due to a trauma I probably experienced in childhood. "See how shallowly you breathe? Your hunched shoulders are a sign of fear."

Three body workers with three interpretations of my body map. One was sadness, a second excessive responsibility, and the third was fear.

So what do my hunched shoulders mean?

Unfortunately, there isn't a "key" that comes with each of our body maps to tell us what the signs and symbols mean. How in the world can we figure out what our bodies are trying to tell us?

Let Your Body Map Be Your Guide

All three of these body workers made the same mistake. They told me what my body map meant according to their theoretical perspective rather than work with me to discern the unique message my body conveyed. While all of these interpretations have merit, and perhaps to some degree or another accurately reflect my situation, none of these body workers knew for sure what my particular body map was saying through my shoulder structure.

A word of caution here—make sure you have a body worker who is open to learning about your body map with you. Take any interpretation given to you by a body worker with a grain of salt. While there may be some principles that guide all of our bodies, only you can know for sure how to read your body map. Your body map uses a personalized set of symbols and the most effective body workers do not assume they know what those symbols may be. Rather, they may give suggestions, offer impressions, and explore options with you about what a particular body signal may mean.

I use the following guidelines to help me understand my body map:

1. My body speaks a unique language and communicates in service of health and wholeness.

2. All body messages have multiple meanings, often relating to a variety of experiences, relationships, and time frames.

3. Only I can say with any certainty what meanings my body map has for me.[1]

An accurate interpretation of our body map will be confirmed through "the 'tingle,' or 'aha' or 'flash,' or 'bell ringing,' or whatever you feel like calling it—the inner knowledge that something is true."[2] Bodyworkers help us explore options and test alternative interpretations, but only we can know for sure what our bodies mean.

In addition to discussing your body map with your body worker, you may want to share your experiences with your talking therapist, support group and friends. All of these trusted people can offer ideas about what your body experiences may mean. Just remember to be cautious of those who claim to know what your body is saying. The means and the ends of body work is trusting our own bodies, because our bodies never lie.

Body Map Principles

Having acknowledged that your body map is unique, I'd like to discuss some general principles common to all body maps. The following may help give you some clues about what your body wants to say to you.

1. Muscle tension and stress

After a workshop I presented on body work and massage, a participant came up to me and said, "I've got intense pain in my hip. What does that mean?"

Some body work perspectives assert that certain feelings or specific messages are carried in particular muscles. For example, it has been said that anger is carried between the shoulder blades or grief carried in the chest area over the heart. As discussed in previous chapters, I believe that feelings are carried in the body, but only you can decide what those feelings may be.

Any feeling can be carried in the muscle tissue, not only stress and tension.For example, I recall one afternoon during my massage training when I volunteered the many large knots in my neck and shoulders for other students to practice their "knot smoothing" techniques. To be honest with you, I didn't really believe that feelings were carried in knots and discarded warnings from the instructor. She had told me that to release too many knots too quickly can result in feeling overwhelmed by the feelings contained.

"I don't buy that," I thought to myself, as I relaxed on the table, glad at last to have the opportunity to have all these sore places ironed out. I went home knot free but woke up the next morning overwhelmed with depression. I met a good friend of mine for brunch. She took one look at me and gasped, "What in the world happened to you! You look horrible."

After thanking her for the review, I explained that nothing bad had happened to me . . . I had ignored my body's pace and inadvertently released more sadness and grief into my system than I was emotionally prepared to face. I was weepy and depressed for several days before I was able to verbally express all the sadness I had too quickly unearthed through touch.

Sadness is one of many feelings that can be held in our muscles. I have experienced a variety of emotions through the release of knots—anger, fear, joy, affection, grief. All of these feelings can be released through body work, and when done so with respect, can take us step by step toward emotional healing. Trust your body to guide you, not only in your interpretation but in the pace in which to proceed. Moving too quickly can release more emotion than can be explored and expressed. Take all the time you need and let your body guide the way.

2. Long-term body structure

Another way our bodies convey messages is through the way we carry ourselves. As I mentioned before, I tend to slouch my shoulders. I've held my body this way for years and, as I've released feelings of shame, sadness, and fear, my posture has improved.

I have benefitted greatly from having my body worker take polaroid pictures of me in a bathing suit from the front, back, and both sides. Together, we talked about the ways I held myself, and what these various postures may mean. I recommend this as a way to gain amazing information about your body map.

These pictures will demonstrate how many of us have "body splits" meaning that we hold one part of our body differently than we do another. Some people have top-bottom splits. These people may have a developed chest but thin, spindly legs. I have strong, thick legs yet carry little weight on my top half.

On the other hand, many people have right-left splits. For example, the picture of my right side looks much younger than the picture of my left side. I actually look like I am a different age, by the way I stand, hold my head, carry my arms. Others I've worked with also have body splits, each carrying a special message about past experiences and current feelings. If you are interested in exploring this in more depth, I recommend reading Bodymind by Ken Dychtwald.[3] While I do not agree with everything this author believes, I find some of his observations worth considering.

As I have discussed previously, another way our bodies carry emotion is through what Carolyn J. Braddock calls, "embodiment styles." She has observed three ways people may respond to childhood trauma, specifically child sexual abuse. These are:

- Rigid:
  - » This body holds muscles firmly, walking heavy on the heels. The breath pattern is irregular, with the breath being held in for a time followed by a heavy sigh. The posture is a stance of aggression and power.
- Collapsed:
  - » This body folds in on itself, with shoulders slumped. Breathing communicates a feeling of "I give up," with shoulders dropping quickly in defeat.
- Inanimate:
  - » Often giving off a feeling like "no one is home," this body style often develops when a person dissociates on a regular basis. This body rarely moves, or makes noise, rather the body offers little resistance or substance. The breath pattern is shallow, with little attention given to events occurring in the present.[4]

I mention this paradigm again because if you identify with these body styles, you may want to explore Carolyn's ideas further in her book, Body Voices.

3.Holding one's breath

The way we breathe tells a lot about how we feel about past or present experiences. Are you aware right now of your breath and what feelings are conveyed?

Often we hold our breath when we are scared or traumatized. If we have a history of terrifying experiences, we may hold our breath as a common practice. Learning to release our breath can unleash a variety of feelings.

Shallow breath may denote weariness, fatigue, sadness, anxiety or hopelessness. Deep sighs may convey rage, grief or loss. Rapid breath may speak of fear, helplessness or rejection. Listen to your breath. What are you saying to yourself? What are the feelings you need to acknowledge and express?

These are but a few ways your body can carry unexpressed emotion, feelings that need to be shared in a safe, mutual relationship in order to be released and healed. As you develop a more trusting relationship with your body worker, the two of you can more personally explore what your feelings and past experiences may be.

Learning to read your body map through body work is a major skill. It requires that we translate the sensations we carry in our bodies into a new language—one that is authentic and effective. For some of us, we are most benefitted by putting our feelings into words. Body workers can help us find the most accurate words to describe these emotions. Once labeled, we can take these feelings to our talking therapists to further explore. Or, we can verbally express them to others in our lives who are able to share our emotional healing.

The Power of Touch

Vimala Schneider McClure was doing a demonstration with a five-month-old baby whose mother massaged her regularly. The mother said that her daughter enjoyed the massage but could not tolerate having her chest touched. McClure asked the mother if the baby had had any trauma to the chest. She learned that the baby had been born two months prematurely and while hospitalized had suffered an injury to the skin that caused some scarring.

During the massage, the baby showed enjoyment at having her legs, feet, and abdomen massaged. When McClure began to stroke her chest, however, the baby cried. Instead of avoiding the chest or quieting the baby, McClure took a deep breath, looked the baby in the eye, and said, "You had a lot of pain. You were so brave. I am listening. Tell me about it."

The baby responded with intense crying. McClure then said, "When you're ready to let go, we'll support you through this. Your mother loves you very much."

The baby looked at McClure intensely while McClure gently massaged her chest. The cries subsided, and the mother picked her up to comfort her.

The next day, when McClure began to massage the baby's chest, the baby opened her arms and smiled.[5]

Every time I hear this story, tears come to my eyes. I know what it is like to be hurt by touch that not only damages physically, but also emotionally and relationally.

But the exciting news is that healing touch can mend past wounds. As I allow someone trustworthy to touch the places that have been hurt, new vistas of health, safety, and intimacy are available to me. My life is being transformed through trusting my body to guide me through the healing power of touch. Confidence replaces insecurity, vitality replaces weariness, and intimacy replaces isolation and shame. Like the baby in this story, the hurt places are soothed by loving, nurturing touch. Memories are discovered and resolved. Feelings are expressed and released. We draw closer to each other as the fear of the past no longer bars our way.

My prayer is that God will guide us all to a deeper experience of wholeness and healing through an increased trust in our bodies. You can trust your body's guidance, your body never lies.

Notes

1 Adapted and modified from Jeremy Taylor's Basic Hints for Dream Work, (Sausalito: Dream Tree Press, 1989).

2 Taylor, 4.

3 Ken Dychtwald, Bodymind, (Los Angeles: Jeremy P. Tarcher, 1986).

4 Carolyn J. Braddock, Body Voices.

5 Laurie Evans, "Impact of Infant Massage on the Neonate and the Parent-Infant Relationship" in Advances in Touch, edited by Nina Gunzenhauser. (NJ: Johnson & Johnson Baby Products Company, 1990), 75.

Author Biography

CARMEN RENEE BERRY

Carmen Renee Berry, M.S.W., M.A., noted author and speaker, is a nationally certified massage technician, social worker and former psychotherapist, who instructs persons of all ages on how to integrate the body into the journey towards wholeness. Ms. Berry promotes healthy lifestyles for stressed and distressed people through her many workshops, seminars, articles and books. She travels extensively speaking to various professional and lay groups.

Ms. Berry is the author of many books including, *When Helping You is Hurting Me; Coming Home to Your Body; Who's to Blame?; girlfriends;* and *The girlfriends Keepsake Book.* Her articles have appeared in *Essence, New Age Journal* and in numerous professional and religious magazines.

Carmen holds an M.S.W. from the University of Southern California's School of Social Work, and an M.A. in Social Sciences from Northern Arizona University. She resides in Pasadena, California.

PageMill Press publishes books in the field of psychology and personal growth. Our authors intend to explore the intellectual, psychological, and spiritual dimensions of our daily lives, such as the mind/body connection, the power of myth and dreams in everyday circumstances, the role of the unconscious in human interactions, and the integration of a fuller experience of the body in life's activities.

We seek to honor the writer's craft by nurturing the interior impulse to create and by producing books that encourage a reader's intellectual and spiritual exploration. We regard highly the collaboration of publisher, editor, and author, with the creative expression that results for readers.

For a catalog of our publications or editorial submissions, please write:

PageMill Press
2716 Ninth Street
Berkeley, CA 94710
PHONE: (510) 848-3600
FAX: (510) 848-1326
E-MAIL: Circulus@aol.com